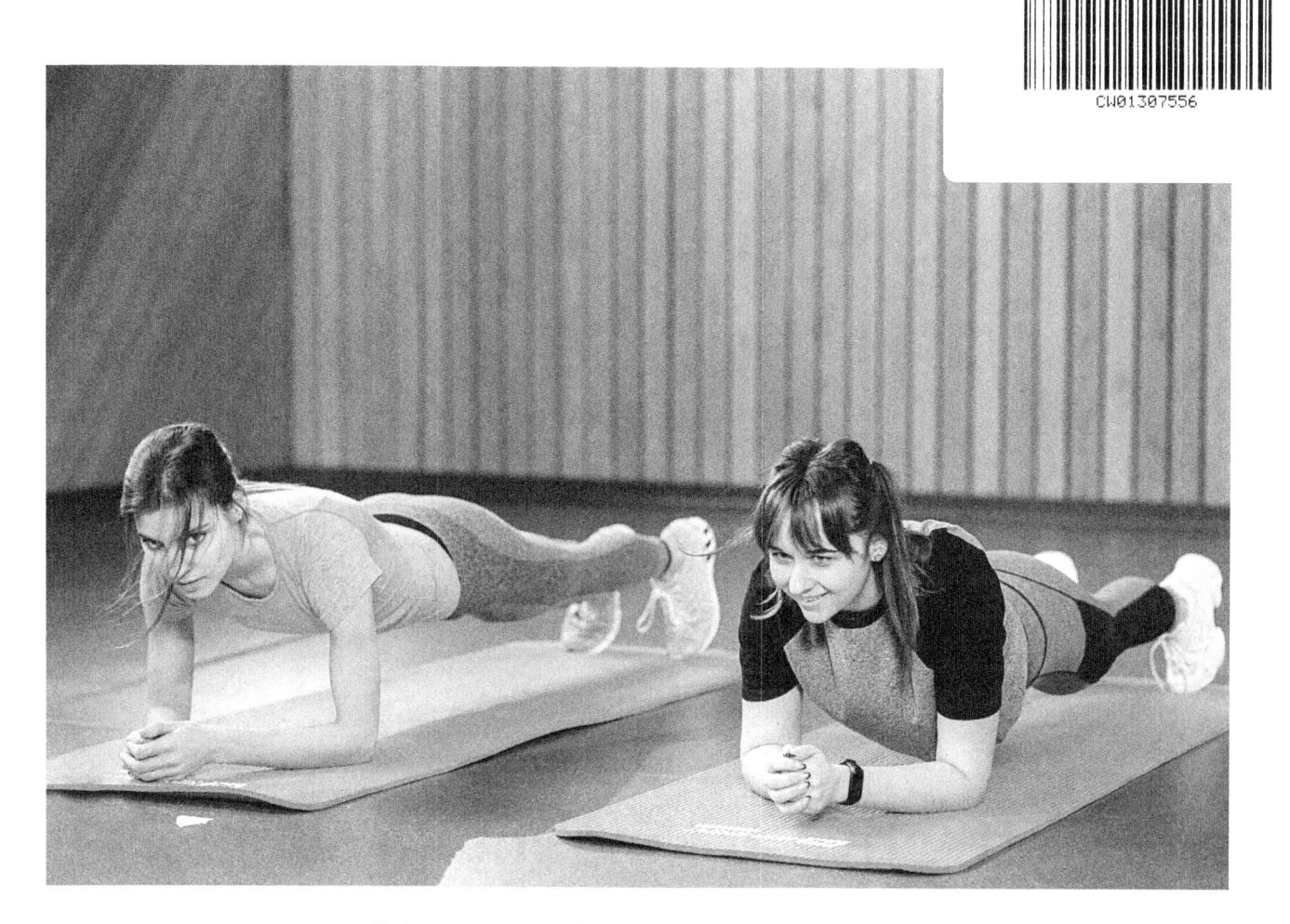

How effective are planks?

Planking consumes more calories, when done consistently, than other center activities like sit-ups. All the more significantly, boards assist with fortifying enormous muscle bunches in your body. Having solid muscles implies you consume more calories, in any event, when you're very still.

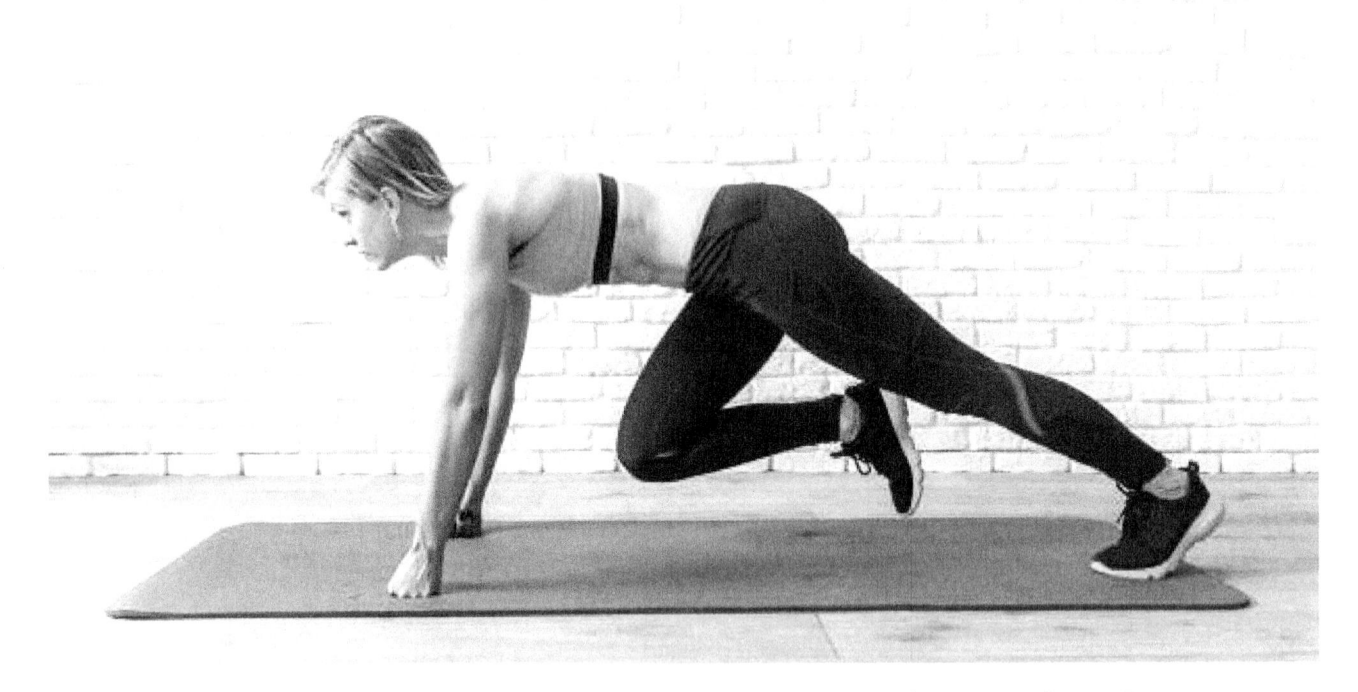

How effective are mountain climbers?

They are unimaginably productive. As a compound activity, hikers work numerous muscle gatherings and joints simultaneously. All in all, they convey serious "value for your money," focusing on center muscles, like back, hips, and abs, as well as glutes, leg muscles, and, surprisingly, your shoulders.

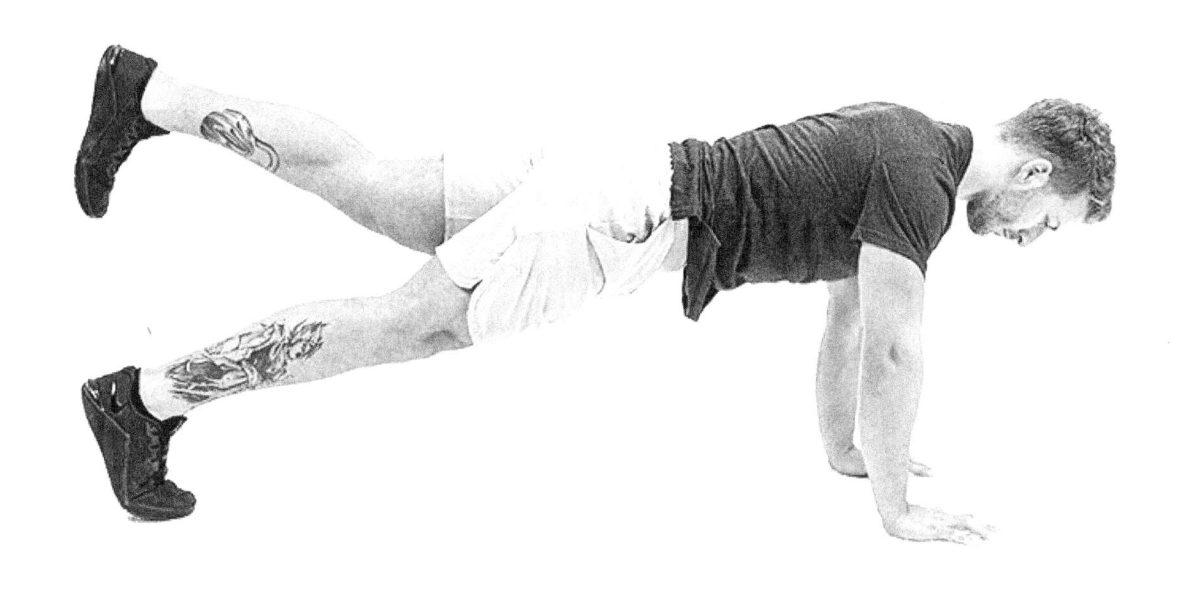

How effective are one-legged push-ups?

The one-leg push-up is a phenomenal compound bodyweight development which fundamentally works the chest muscles. However, the rear arm muscles and front deltoids likewise get excitement as optional movers during the activity. Lifting one leg works on your equilibrium and furthermore works stabilizer muscles giving a utilitarian advantage.

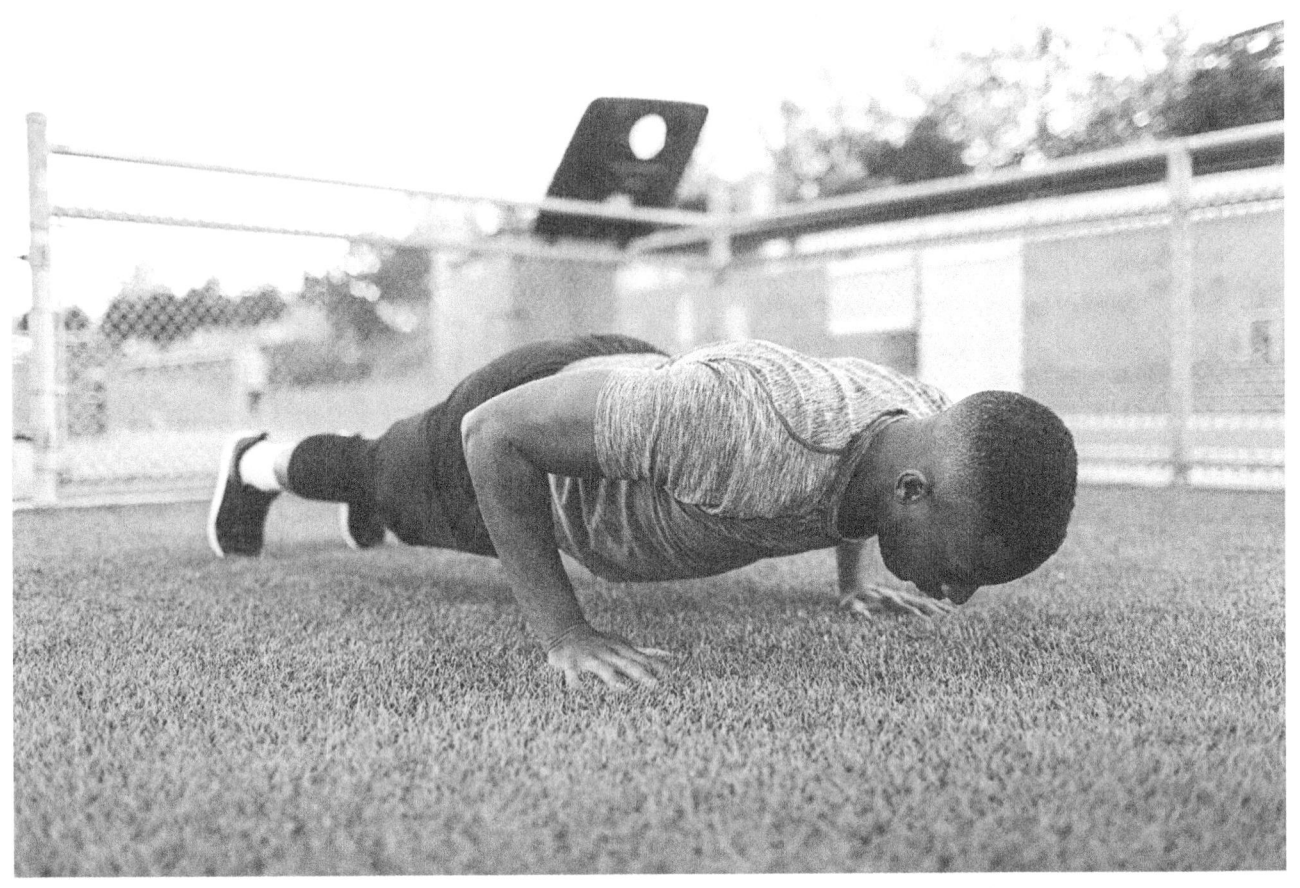

How effective are push-ups?

Traditional pushups are beneficial for building upper body strength. They work the triceps, pectoral muscles, and shoulders. When done with proper form, they can also strengthen the lower back and core by engaging (pulling in) the abdominal muscles. Pushups are a fast and effective exercise for building strength.

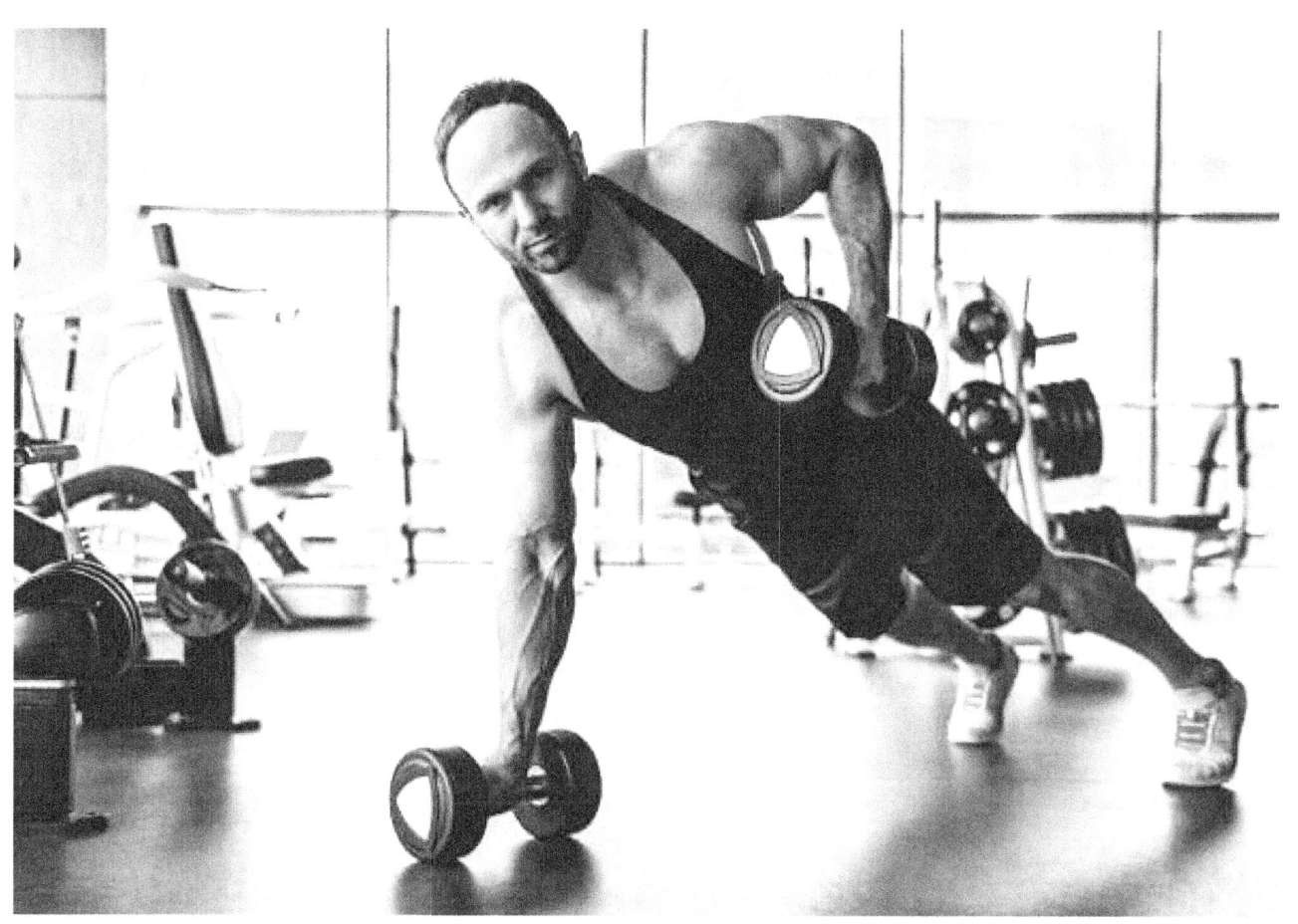

How effective are push-ups with rotation

Push up with turn is a useful preparation practice that coordinates two mainstays of regular human development: pushing/pulling and pivot. it works the muscles of the chest, foremost deltoid and rear arm muscles while requesting the adjustment strength of both shoulder bones and spine.

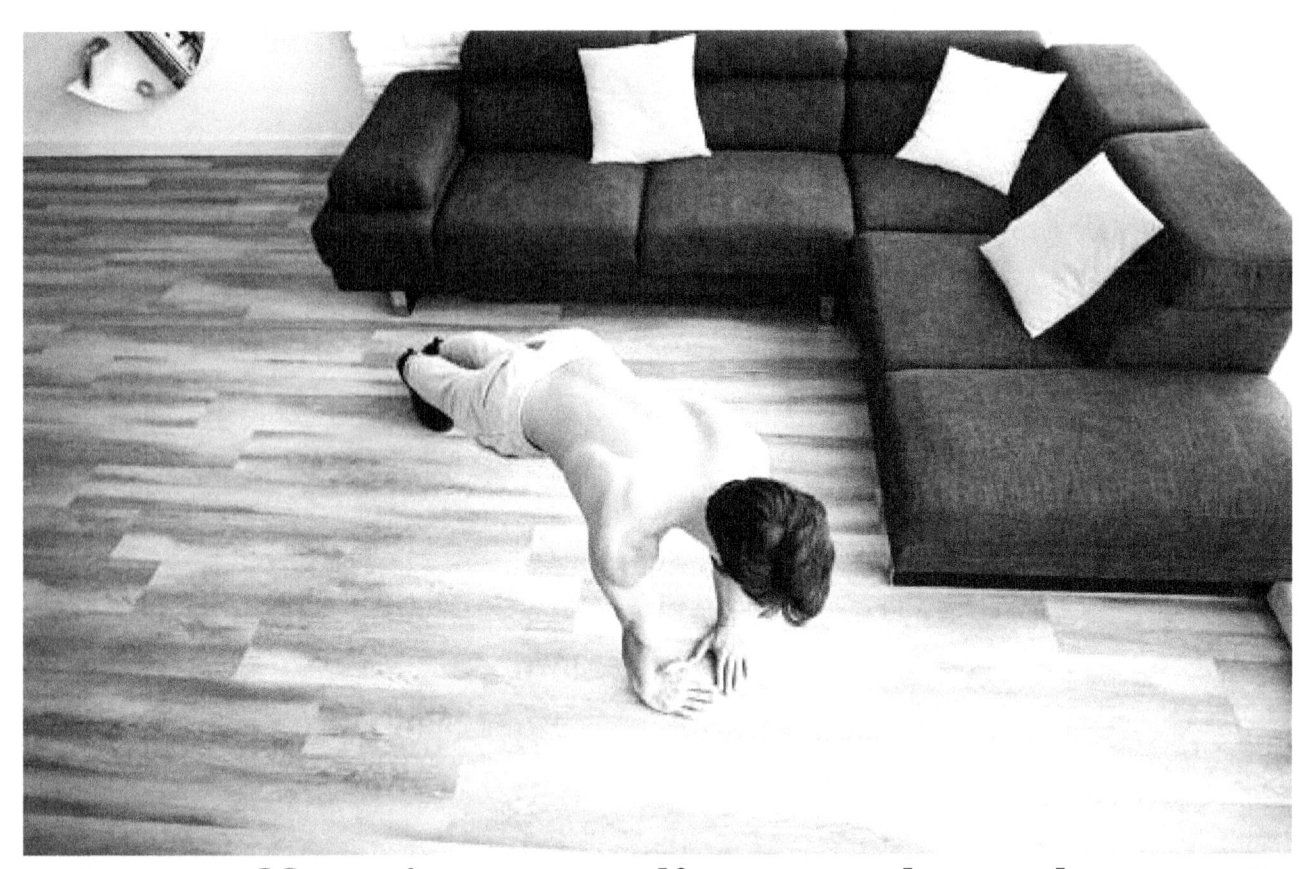

How effective are diamond push-ups?

The jewel push-up is one of the best rear arm muscles works out. The extraordinary hand position of this bodyweight practice enacts your rear arm muscles brachii in excess of a standard push-up.

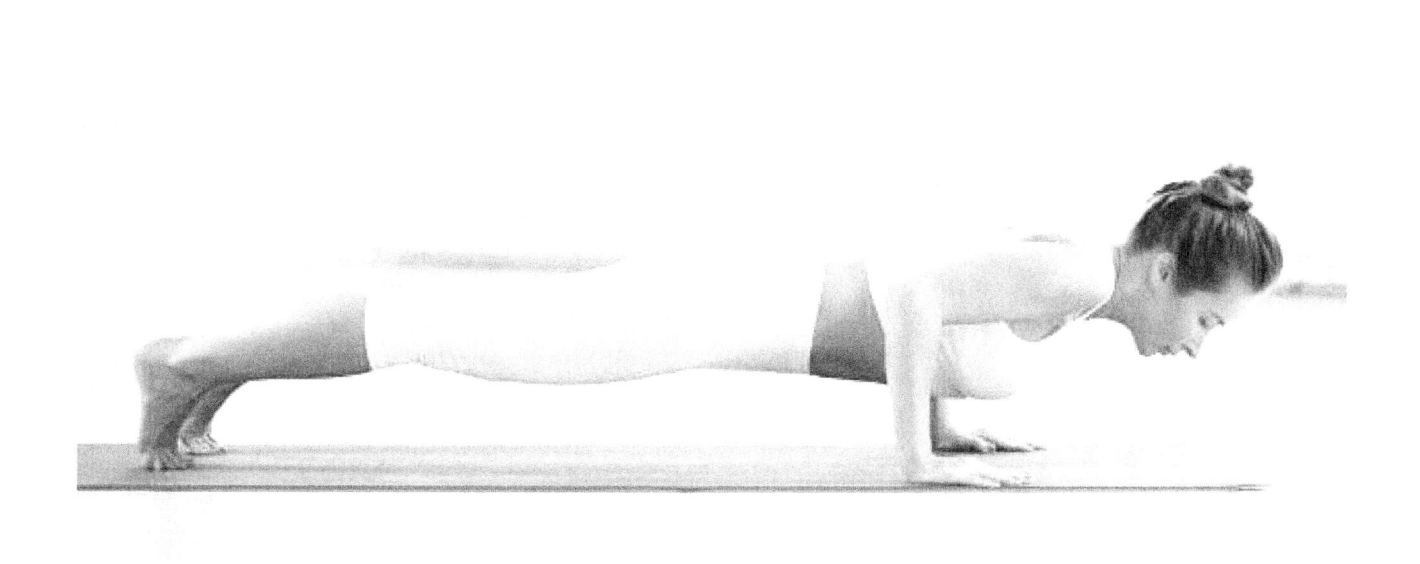

How effective are chaturanga push-ups?

Chaturanga Varieties and Advantages
This is perhaps of the most difficult posture in the fundamental progression of a Vinyasa class, says Peterson. It's an extraordinary move for developing your chest area fortitude, and you'll feel it in your chest, shoulders, back, rear arm muscles, biceps, and lower arms.

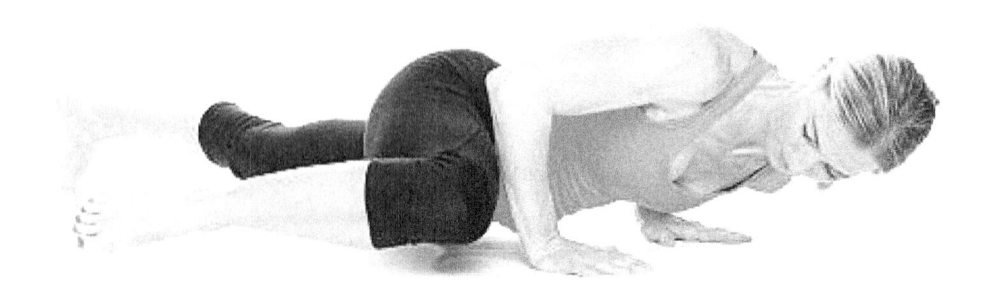

How effective are spiderman push-ups?

Spiderman push-ups build strength throughout your upper body, especially in your triceps, forearms, deltoids, and upper pecs. 3. Spiderman push-ups can improve core strength and stability. As you lift your leg during the exercise, you activate core muscles to stabilize yourself more than a regular push-up.

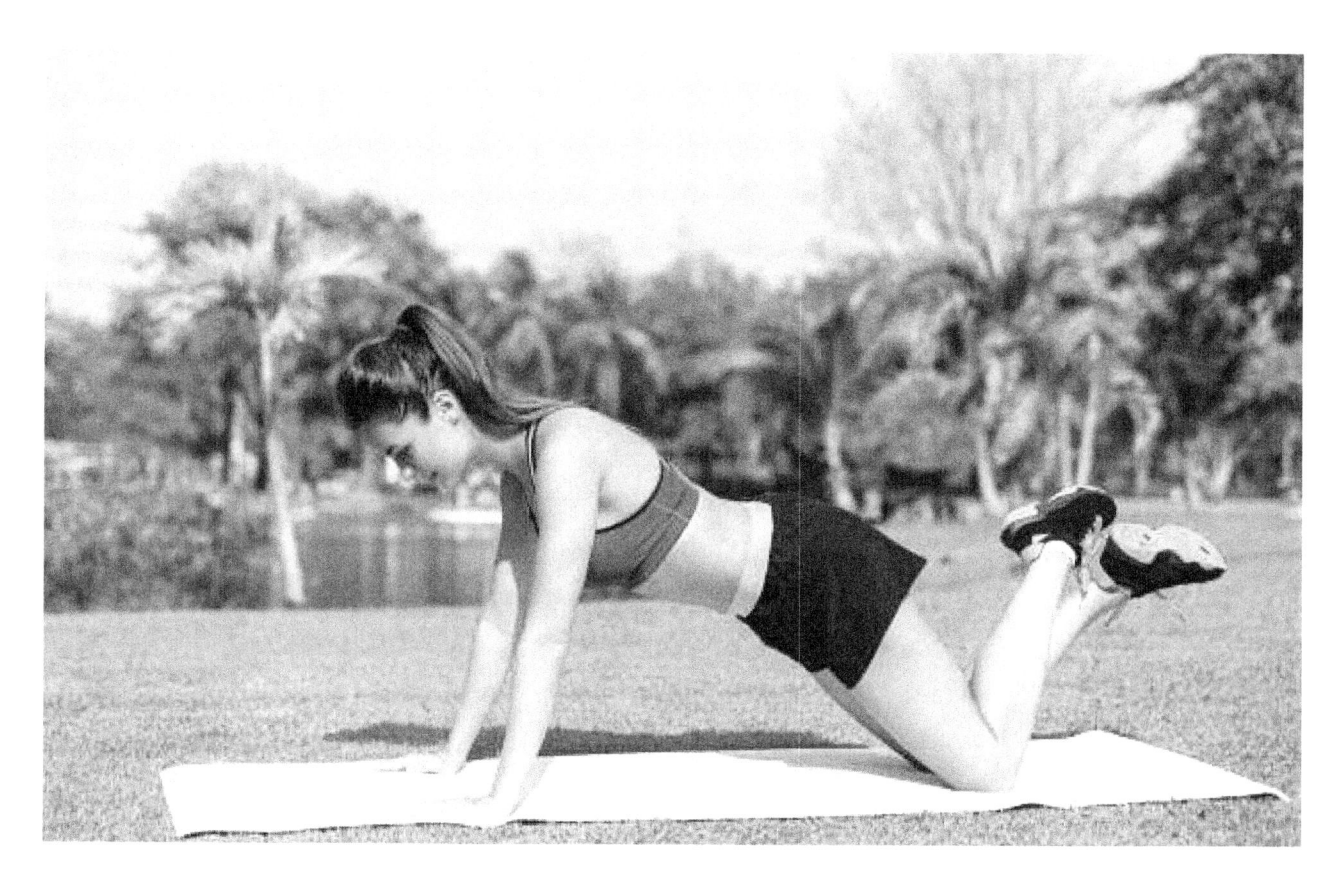

How are effective are asymmetrical push-ups?

There's a well established demeanor that knee push-ups give no genuine advantage to developing chest area fortitude, however late discoveries show this is unwarranted and false. Specialists say knee push-ups can be extremely useful and share a few top ways to make them work for you.

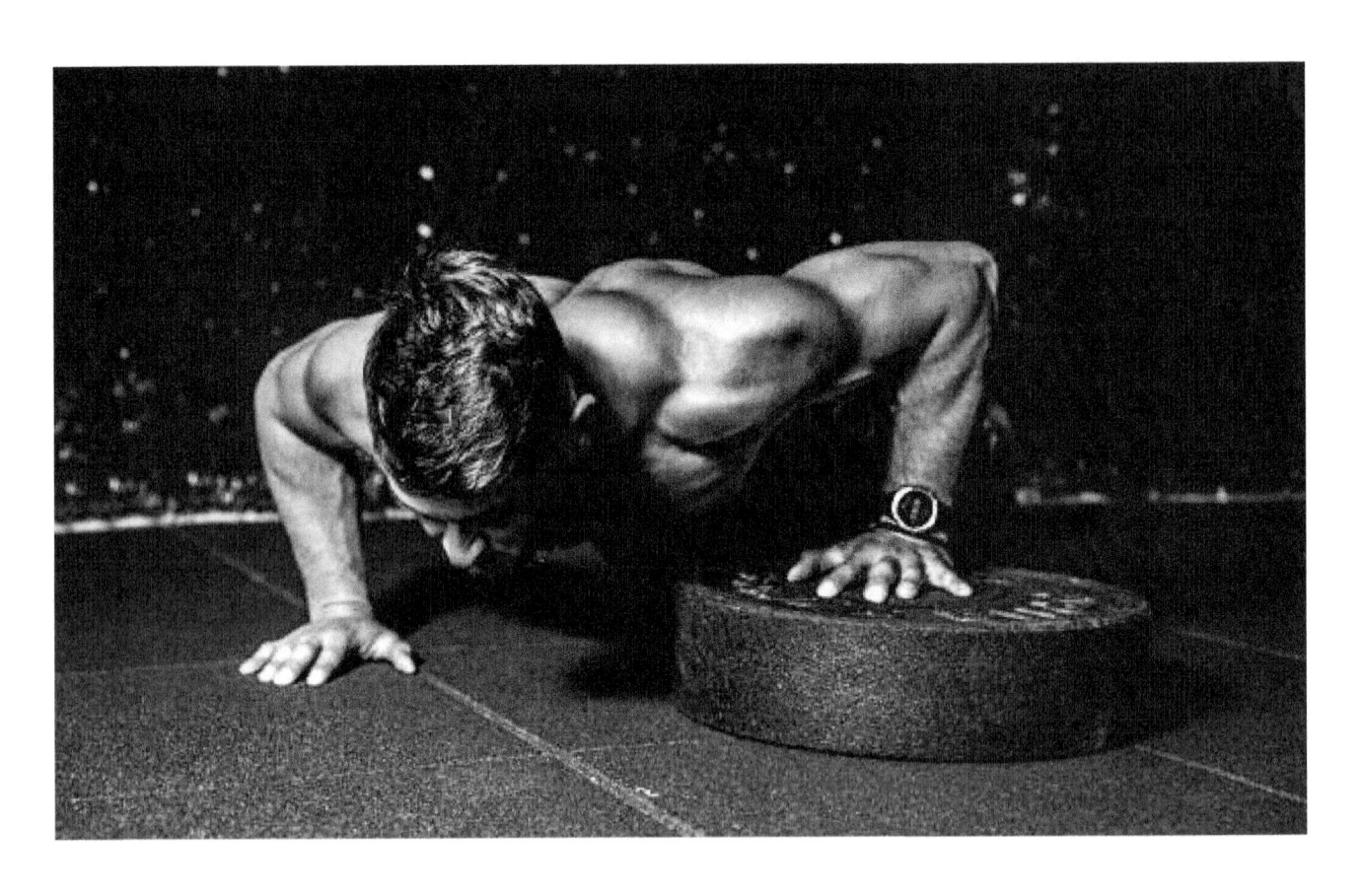

How effective are uneven push-ups?

Alternating Uneven Push-Ups are an advanced variation of the basic push-up. They provide a more rigorous workout by engaging stability muscle groups that are not normally engaged during a regular push-up. Also, uneven push-ups trick your body into going all the way down, giving you the full motion of the push-up.

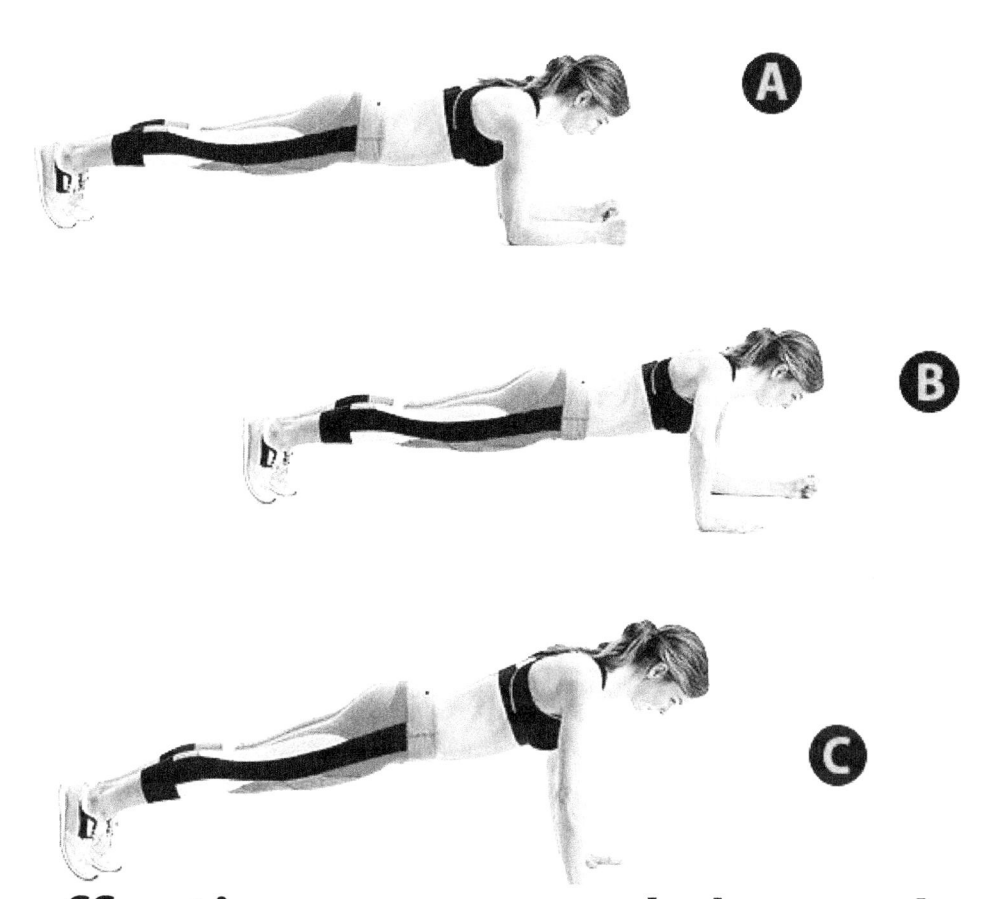

How effective are up-and-down planks?

The all over board fortifies and tones your center, glutes, arms, wrists, and shoulders. This exercise assists with working on your stance, fixes the waist, and lifts weight reduction.

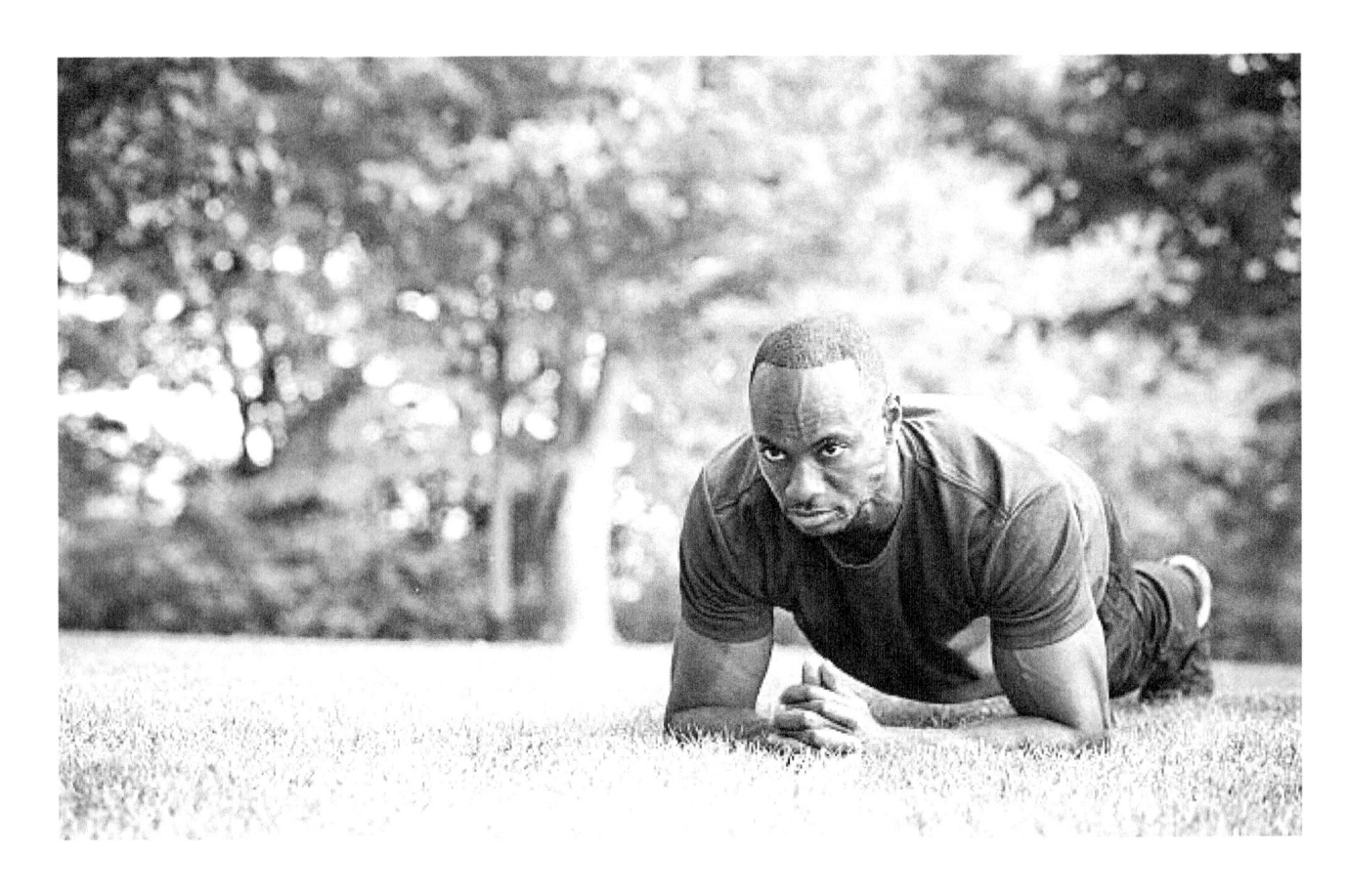

How effective are elbow planks?

Boards on your elbows are best for focusing on the center muscles. Being more level to the floor implies your center needs to work harder to keep you stable. You can build the accentuation on the obliques and rectus abdominis much more by putting your lower arms on a temperamental surface, for example, an activity ball.

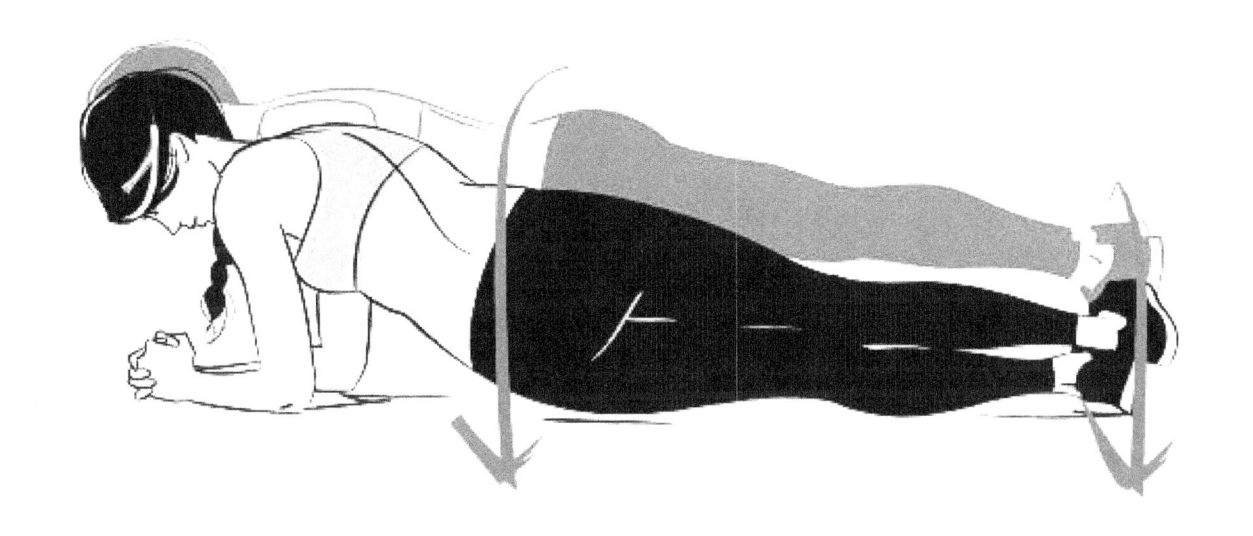

How effective are plank hip dips?

This exercise fortifies your abs, obliques, and lower back, and assists with managing down your midriff. It likewise upgrades the adaptability of your spine and can assist with working on your equilibrium, soundness, and stance.

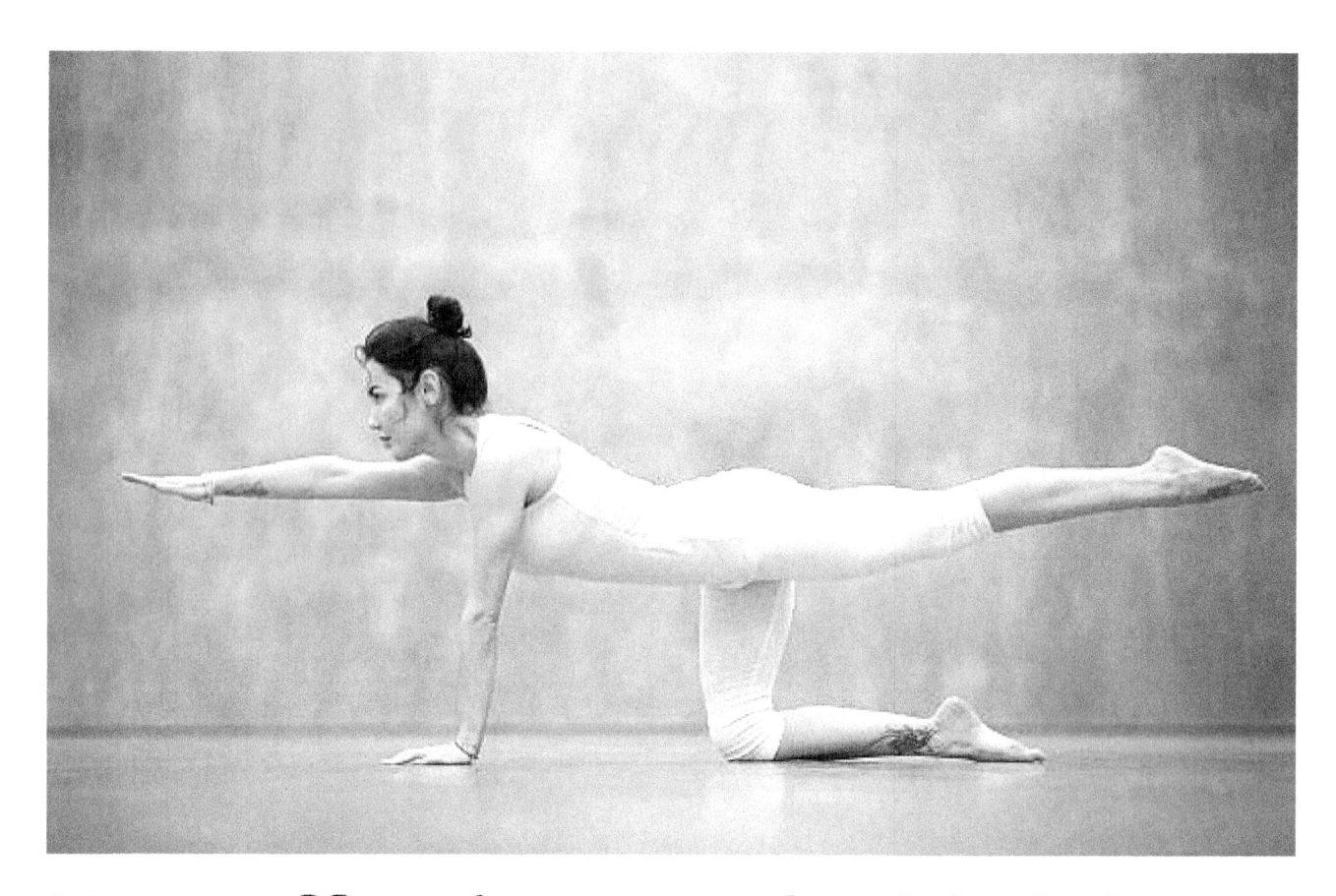

How effective are the bird dogs?

The bird dog is a basic center activity that further develops dependability, supports an unbiased spine, and eases low back torment. This exercise present purposes the entire body to target and fortify your center, hips, and back muscles. It likewise advances legitimate stance and increment scope of movement.

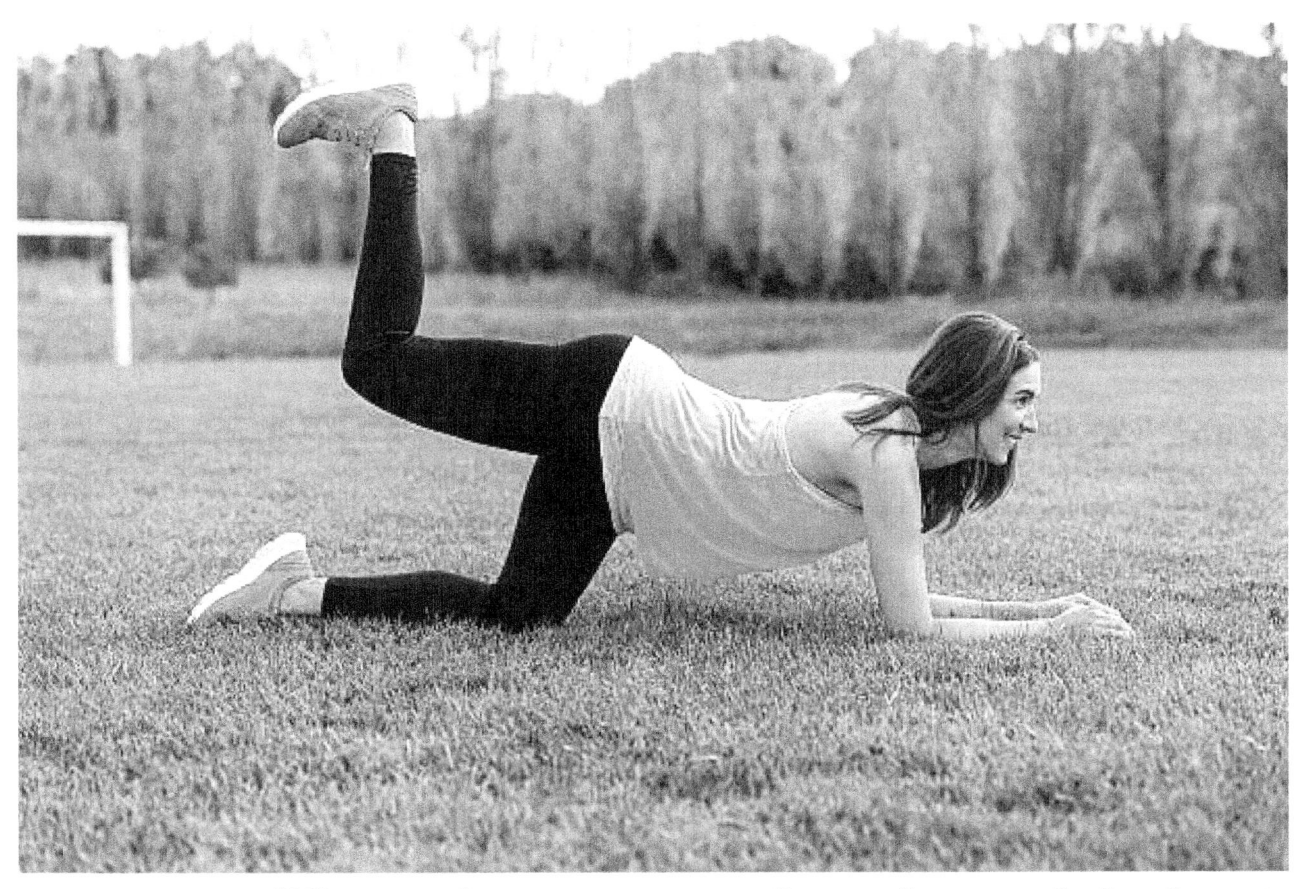

How effective are donkey kicks?

Donkey kicks are perfect for both security and conditioning, Beam says. They focus on your gluteus maximus — the biggest of your three glutes muscles, and the main part of your goods. They likewise work your center and shoulder muscles, since your whole body needs to stay stable while your leg lifts

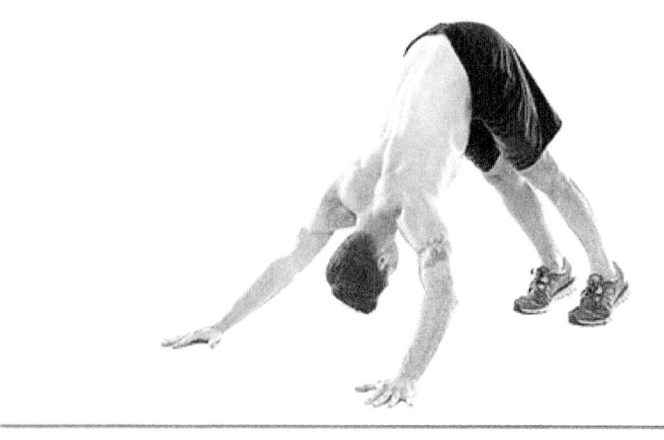

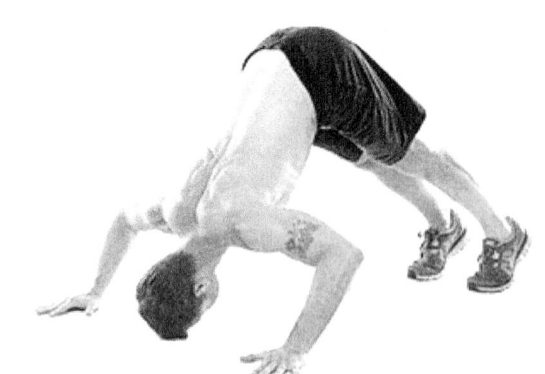

How effective are down dog push-ups?

What Muscles Does A Downward Dog Push Up Work? Downward Dog Push Up is a magnificent chest area move that works your chest, back, shoulders, arms and, surprisingly, your center! Downward Dog Push Up is likewise an extraordinary method for getting a stretch for the whole posterior of your body.

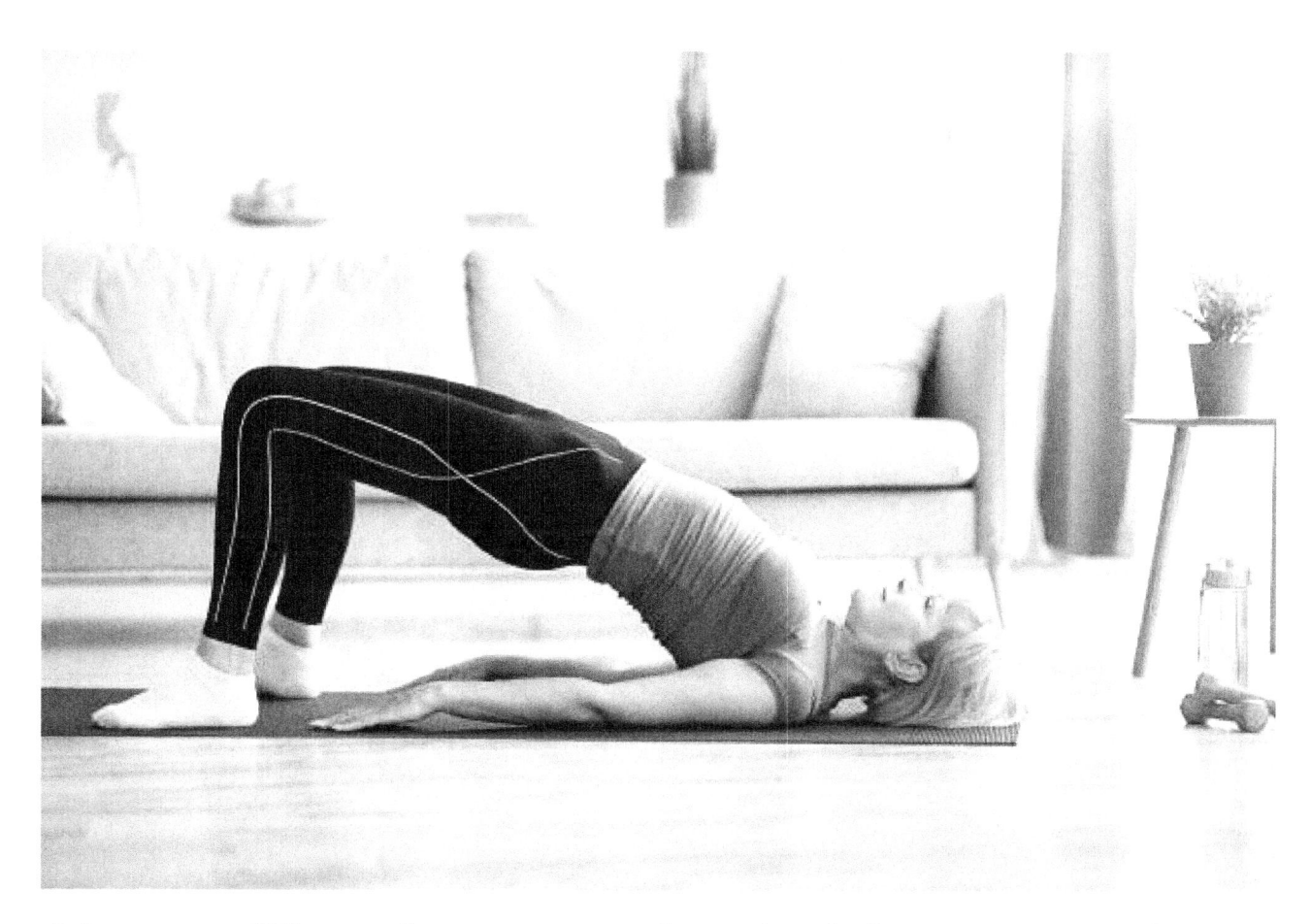

How effective are the bridge exercise?

The bridge exercise is the ideal expansion to an at-home exercise as it requires no hardware and insignificant space. It's a decent activity for hip versatility and reinforcing the lower back, and as it's low-influence, extraordinary for anybody has knee or hip worries.

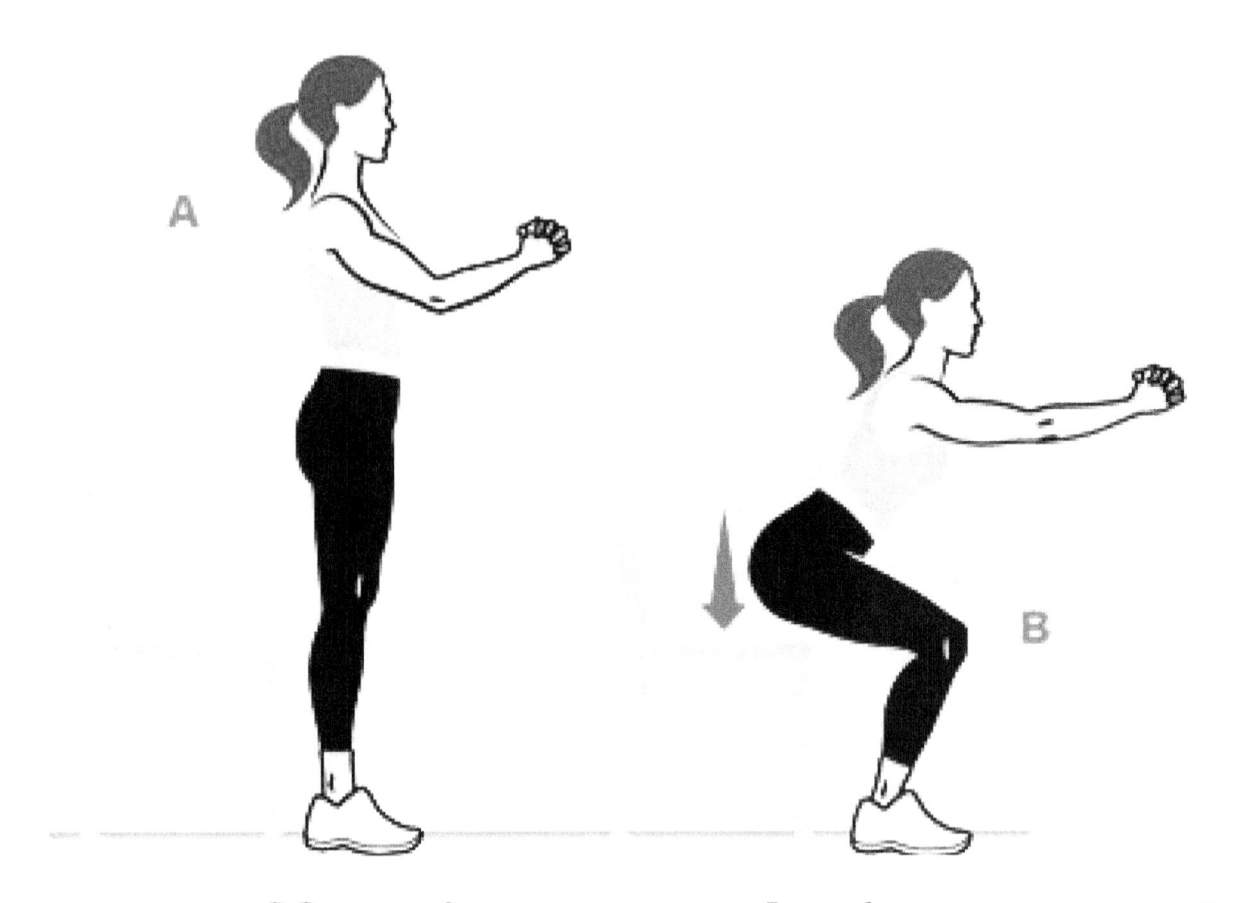

How effective are chair squats?

Seat squats are an extraordinary method for developing the fortitude in your leg muscles in the event that you're new to working out. The seat offers added help as you work your glutes, hamstrings, and quads.

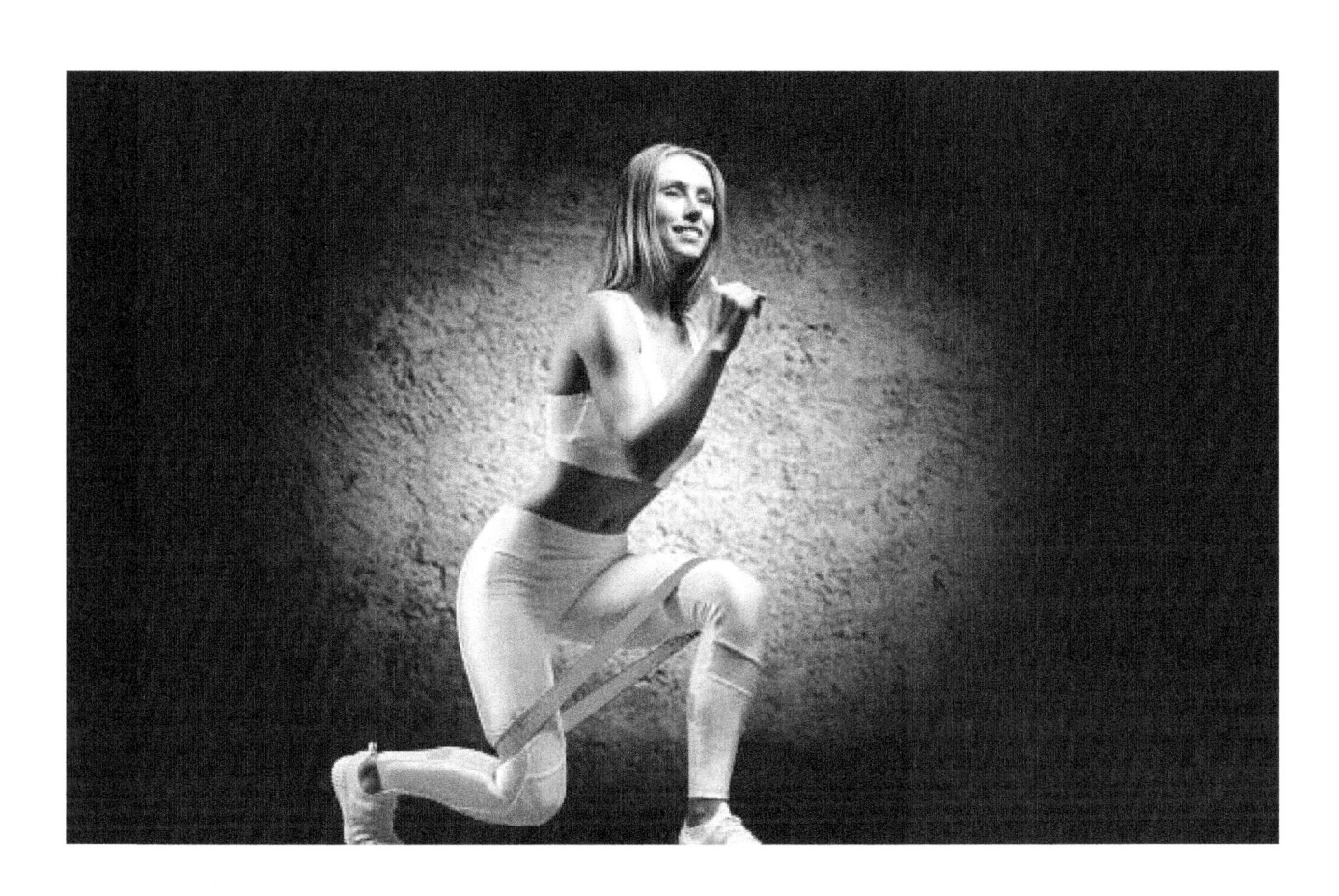

How effective are stationary lunges?

Fixed Lunges work essentially every lower body muscle including your glutes, quads, hamstrings and calves. They're an extraordinary move to consolidate in your lower body exercises and they require zero hardware — simply your own bodyweight!

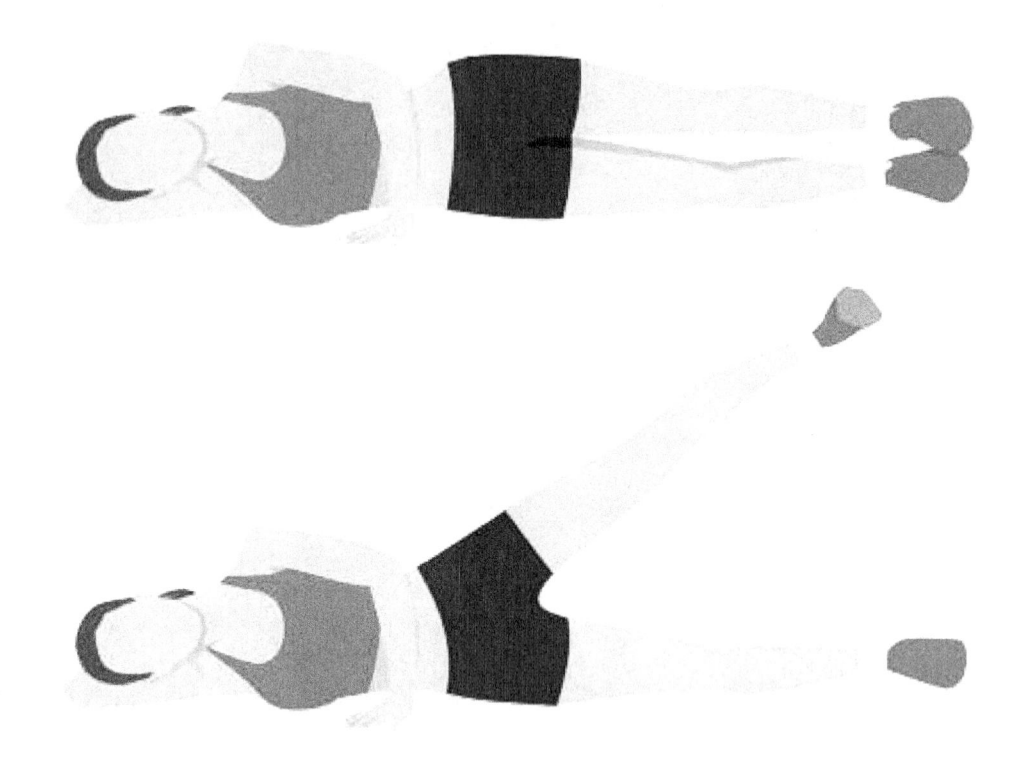

How effective are side-lying hip abduction?

Advantages of the Side-Lying Hip Abduction

The side-lying hip snatching is one of the most incredible activities for working the gluteus medius. 1 It likewise actuates the gluteus medius and tensor fasciae latae (external thigh). These muscles raise the leg horizontally away from the body and turn the leg outward.

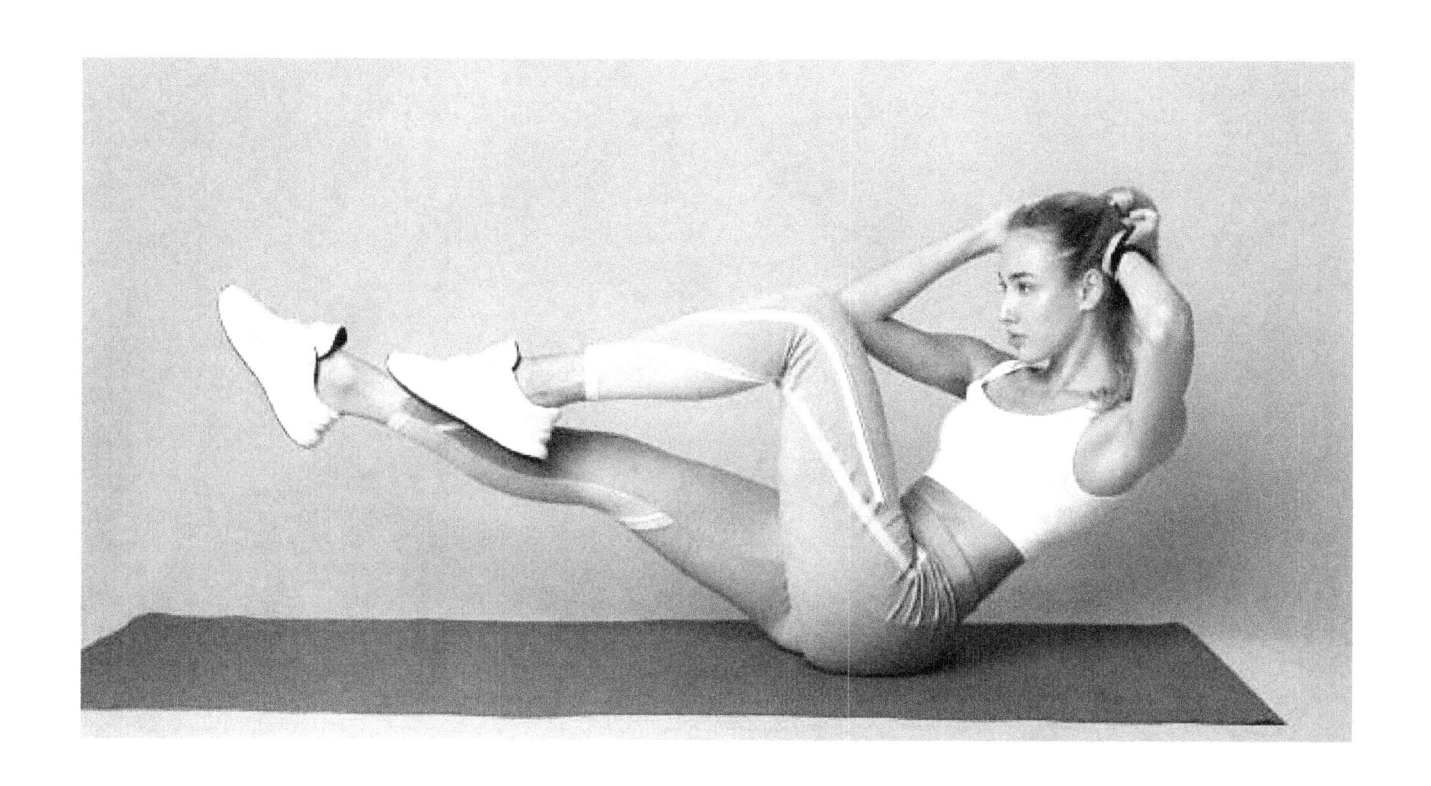

How effective are bicycle crunches?

The bike crunch is a powerful stomach muscle work out, arriving at the typical abs as well as the profound abs and the obliques. 1 to work your center, this air bike move is an extraordinary decision. It's a no-hardware, fledgling's activity you can do anyplace.

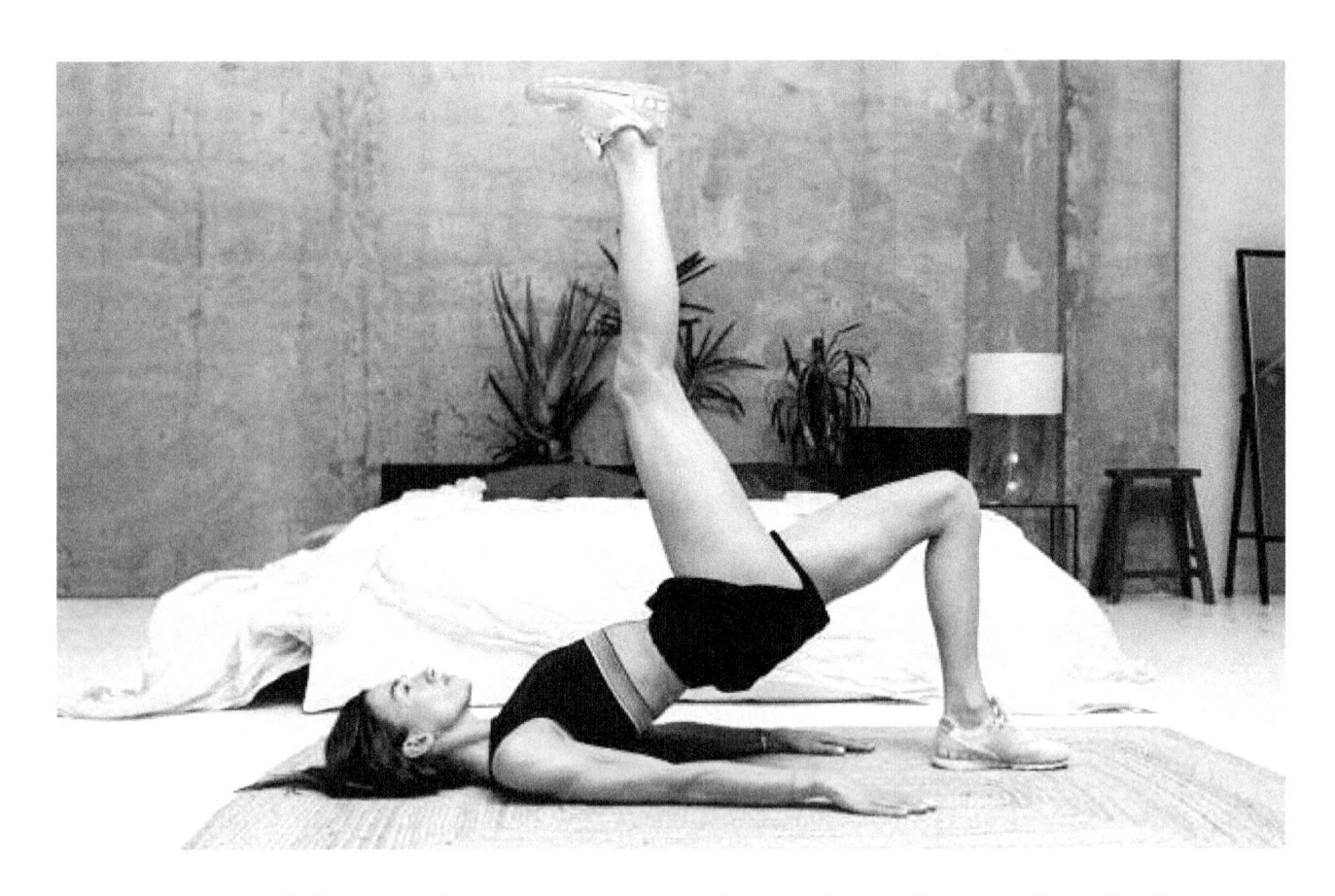

How effective are single-leg bridge?

The single leg bridge exercise is an extraordinary method for disconnecting and reinforce the hip extensors (glutes and hamstrings). Since it doesn't need hardware, this exercise squeezes into a lower body strength exercise performed at the rec center, at home, or even while voyaging.

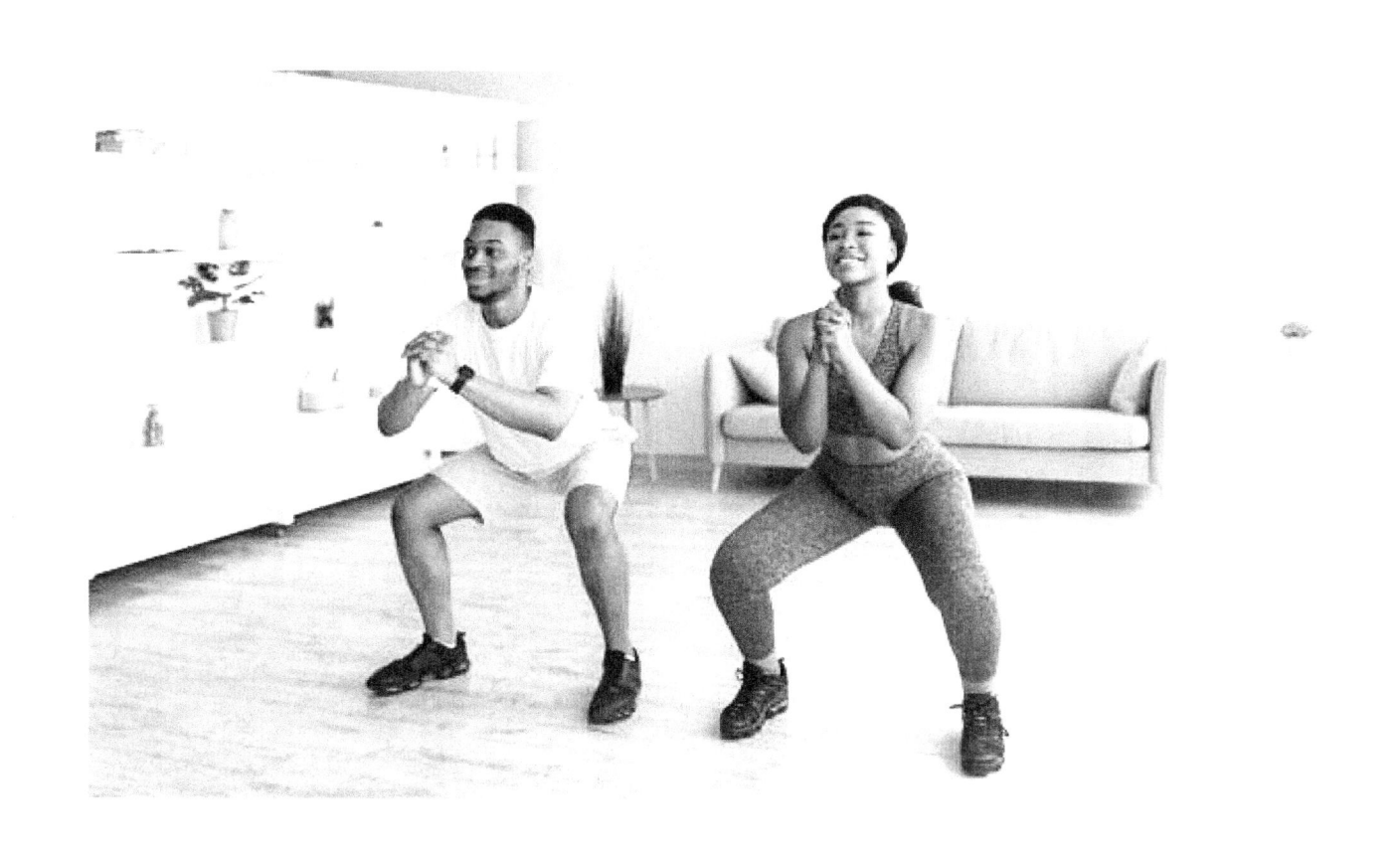

How effective are squats?
Squats consume calories and could assist you with getting thinner. They likewise bring down your possibilities harming your knees and lower legs. As you work out, the development fortifies your ligaments, bones, and tendons around the leg muscles.

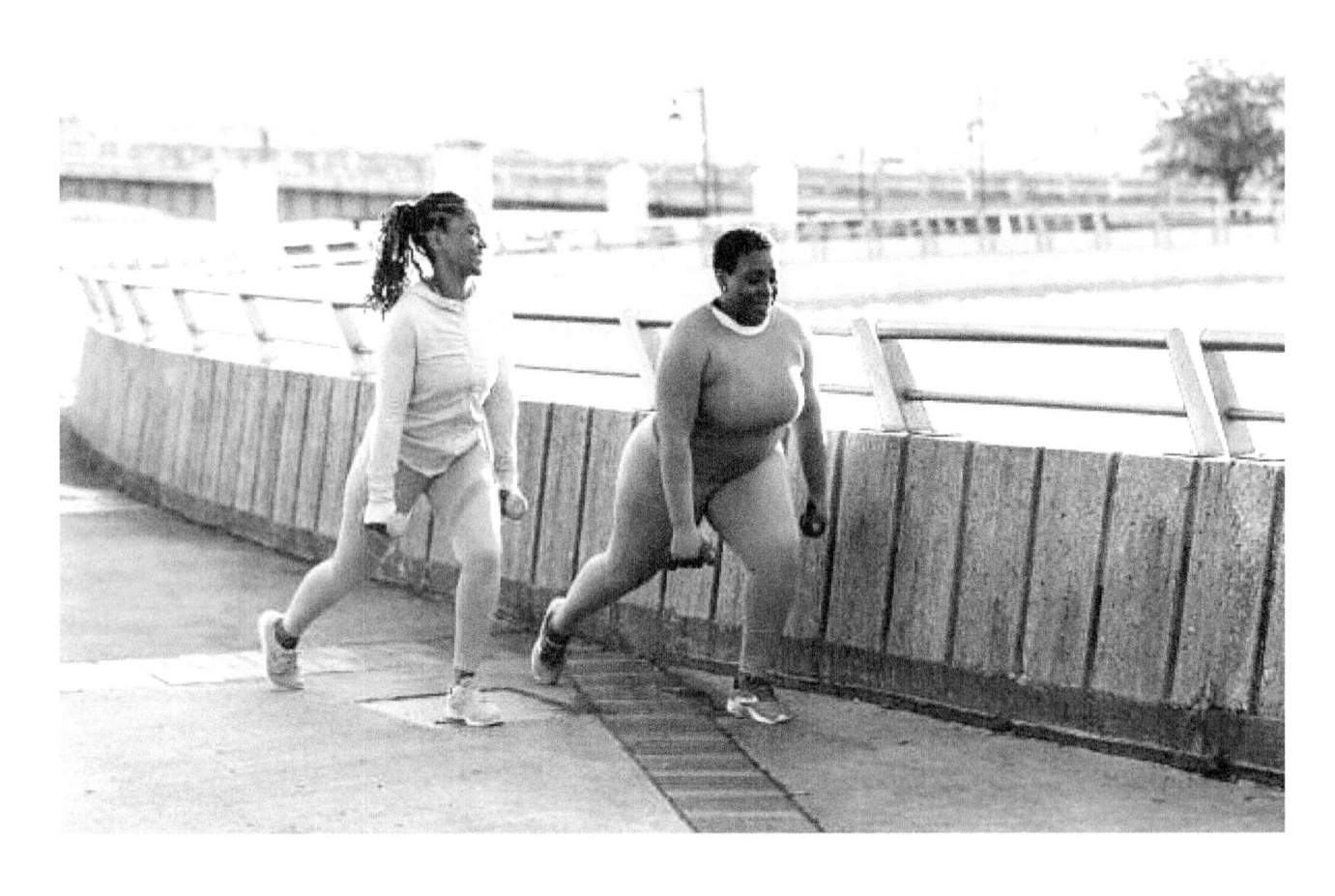

How effective are walking lunges?

Walking lunges can assist with expanding your scope of movement by assisting with expanding adaptability, and relax your hips and hamstrings. This can assist with further developing stance and equilibrium, which can be gainful to competitors, easygoing exercisers, and wellness fledglings the same.

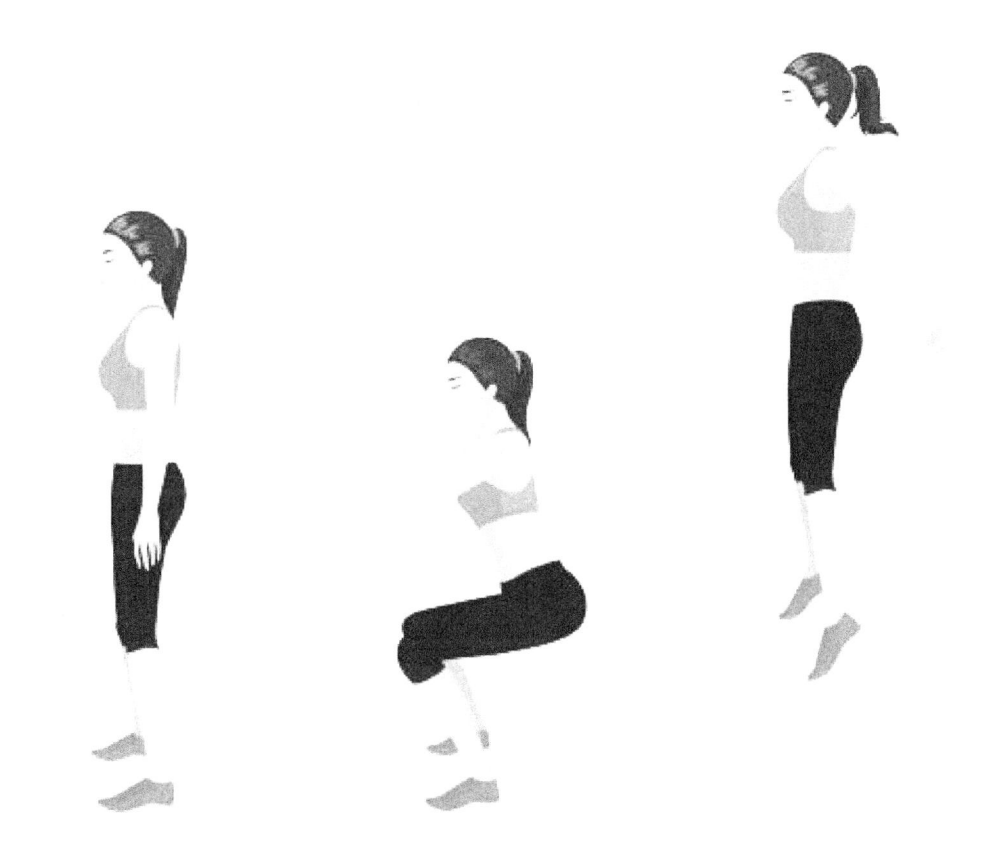

How effective are jump squats?

The jump squat is a stellar method for working your glutes, quads, hips, and hamstrings. Since it gives both strength preparing and cardiovascular advantages, it's a heavenly piece of a balanced exercise. Simply make a point to consummate your structure first. In the event that you have knee, hip, or lower leg probs, avoiding this one is ideal.

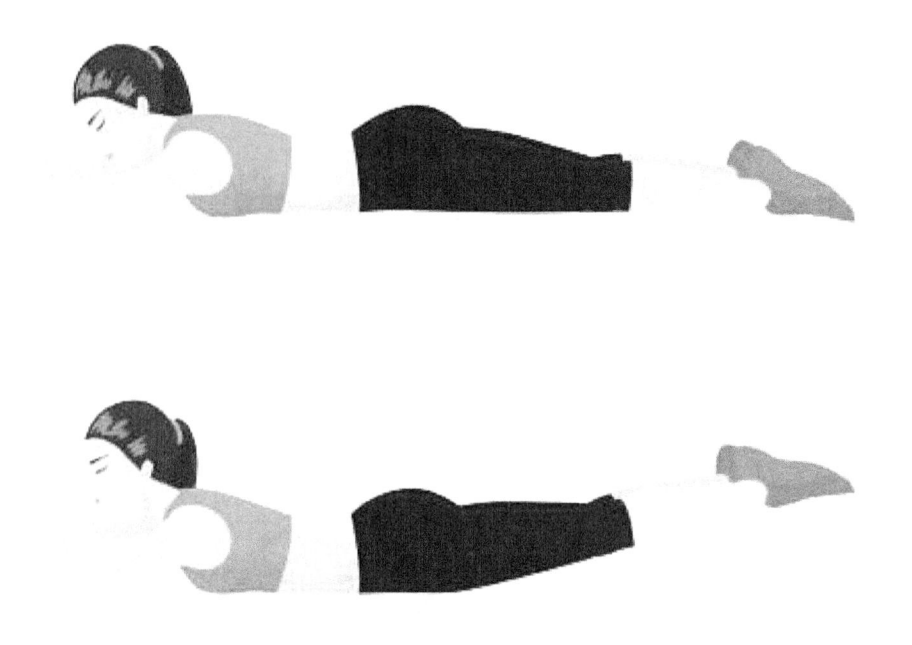

How effective is the superman exercise?

The superman exercise is a powerful and proficient activity for individuals of all wellness levels. It focuses on your lower back muscles, glutes, hamstrings, and abs. Furthermore, it supplements other center activities —, for example, leg raises and situps — that for the most part center around the stomach muscles toward the front of your body.

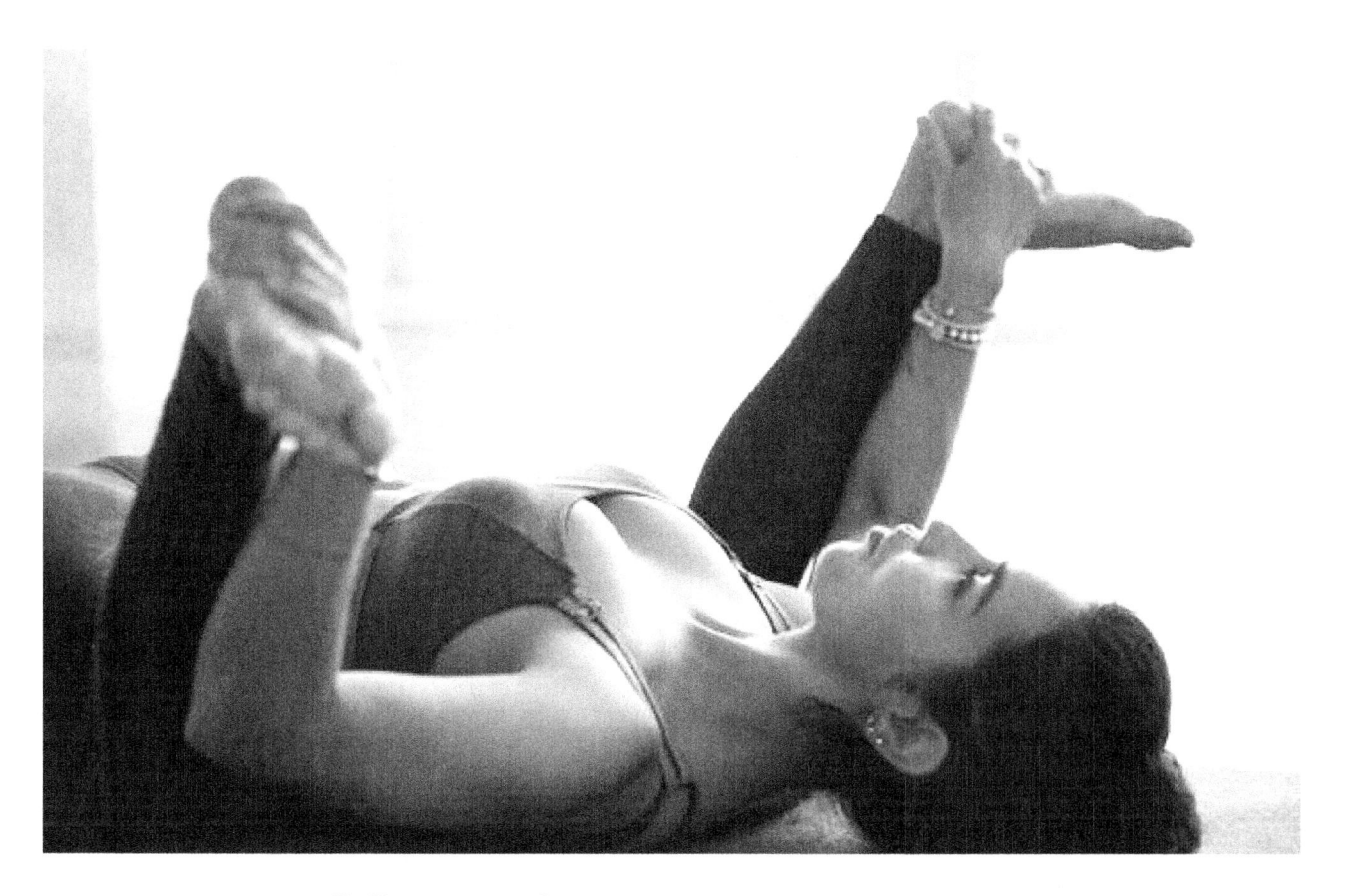

How effective are dead bug?

The dead bug exercise is a protected and powerful method for reinforcing and balance out your center, spine, and back muscles. This works on your stance and eases and forestall low back torment. You'll likewise further develop equilibrium and coordination.

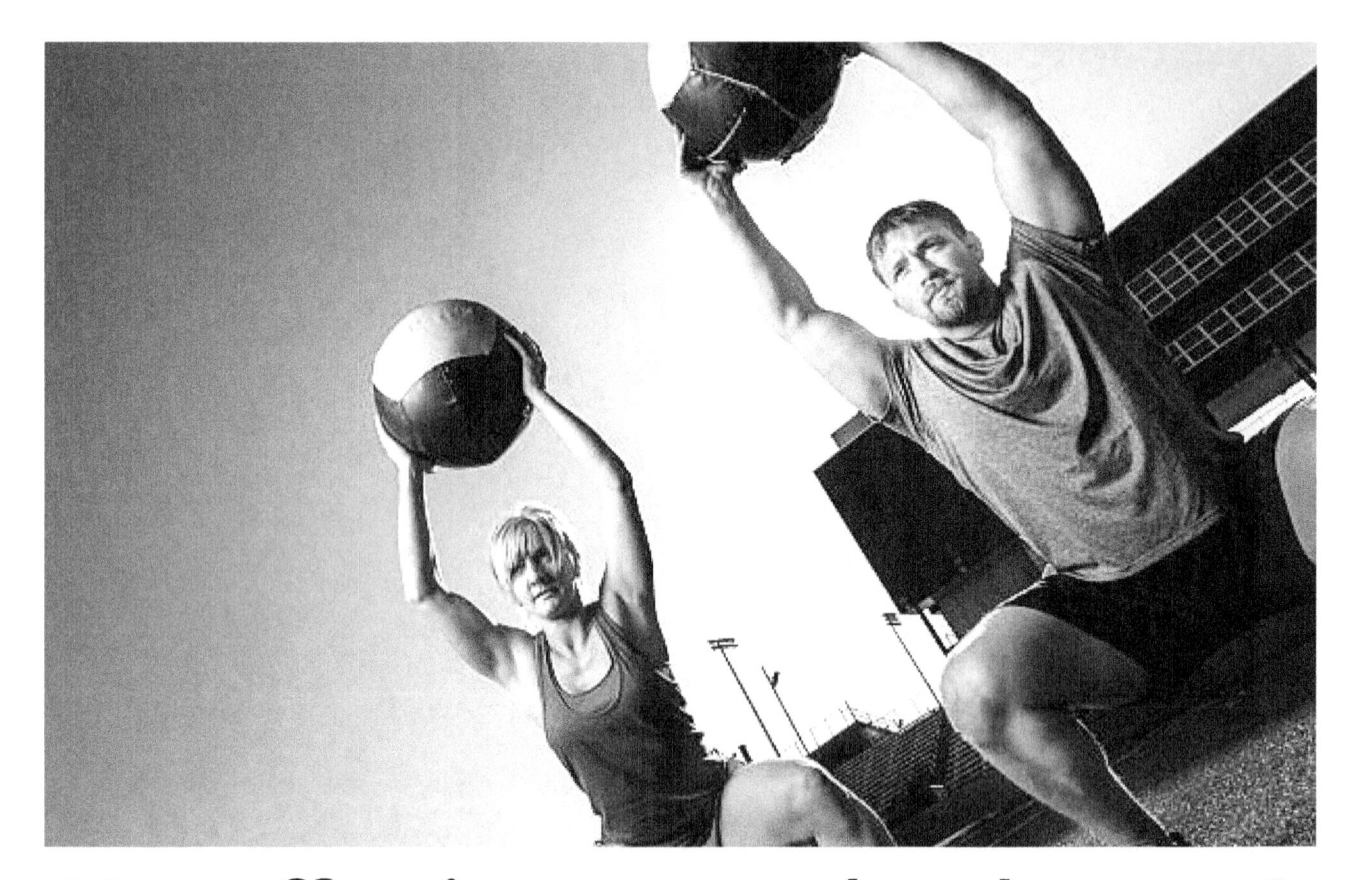

How effective are overhead squats?

Overhead squats can increase your overall strength. The overhead squat activates muscles in your upper body like your triceps and deltoids, as well as muscles in your lower body—including your hamstrings, adductors, quadriceps, and lower back muscles.

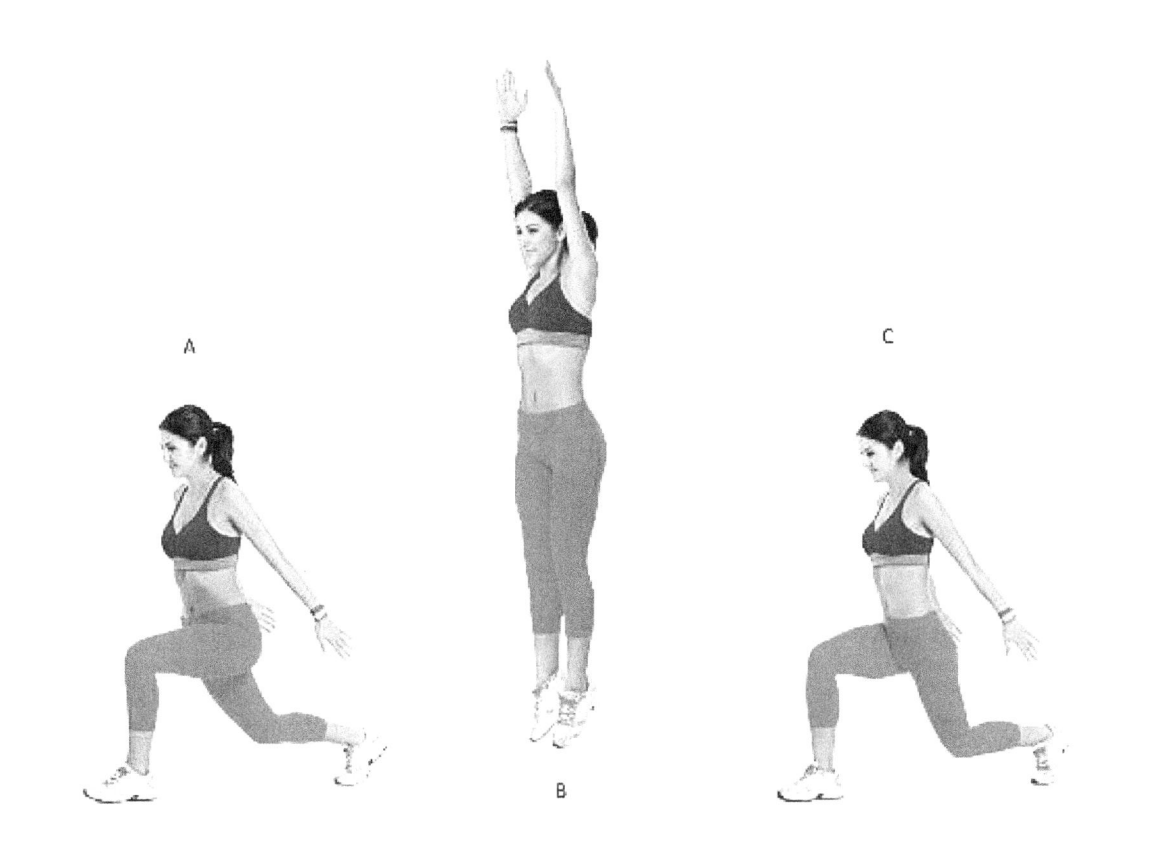

How effective are jumping lunges?

Jumping lunges are a fabulous lower body practice that builds the power and trouble of the essential lunge by adding a leap. The expansion of a plyometric hop not just difficulties the quads, hamstrings, glutes, hip flexors, and calves, yet it likewise enlists your cardiovascular framework.

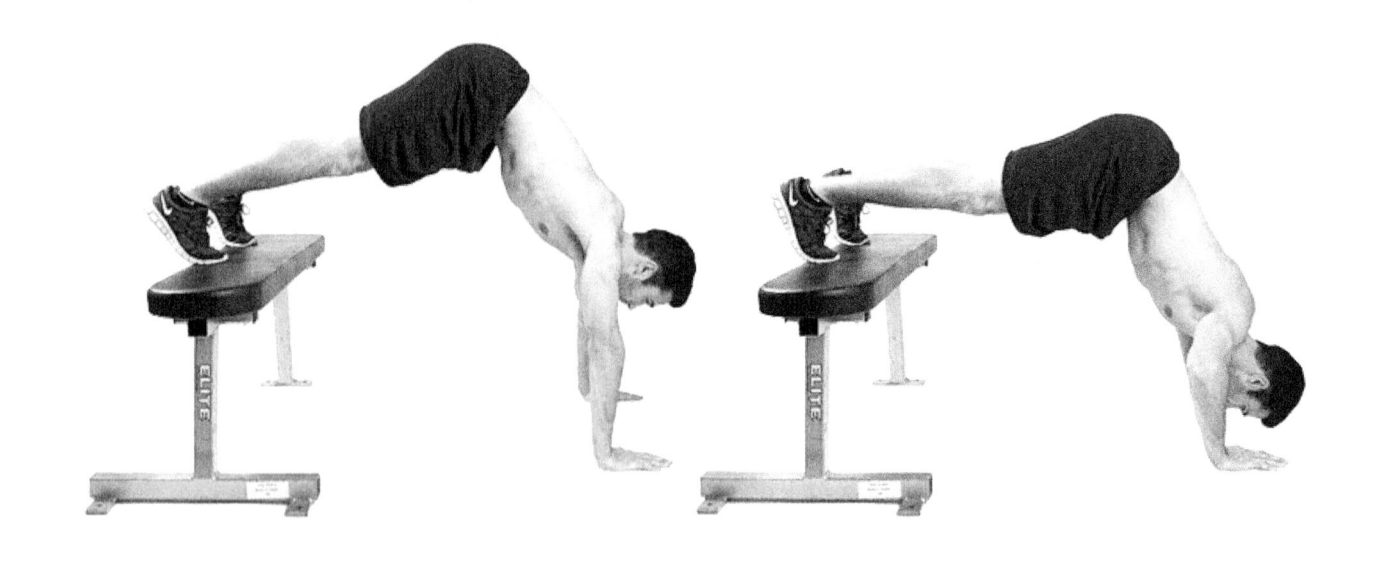

How effective are elevated pike push-ups?

The Foot Raised Pike Push-Up is an extraordinary bodyweight exercise to serious areas of strength for foster. In the event that you're hoping to develop the fortitude expected for handstand push-ups, this drill is ideally suited for you. The main hardware you'll require is an item to lift your feet.

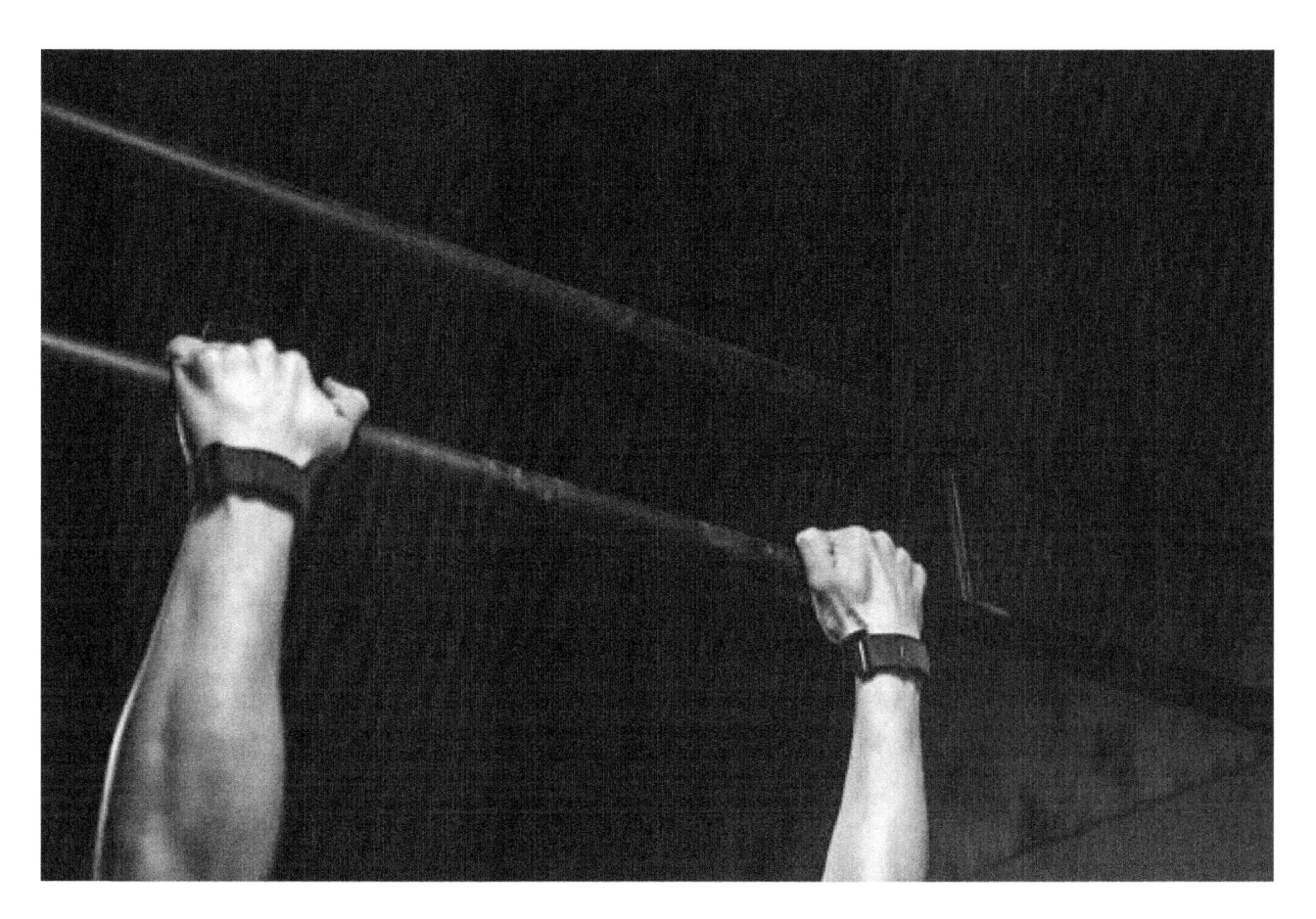

How effective are hollow holds?

The hollow hold fortifies the muscles that settle your lower back during athletic and ordinary developments. Uniformly fortified glutes, hip flexors, and abs assist with keeping your spine in appropriate arrangement and stay away from pressure to the vertebrae and circles.

BURPEE

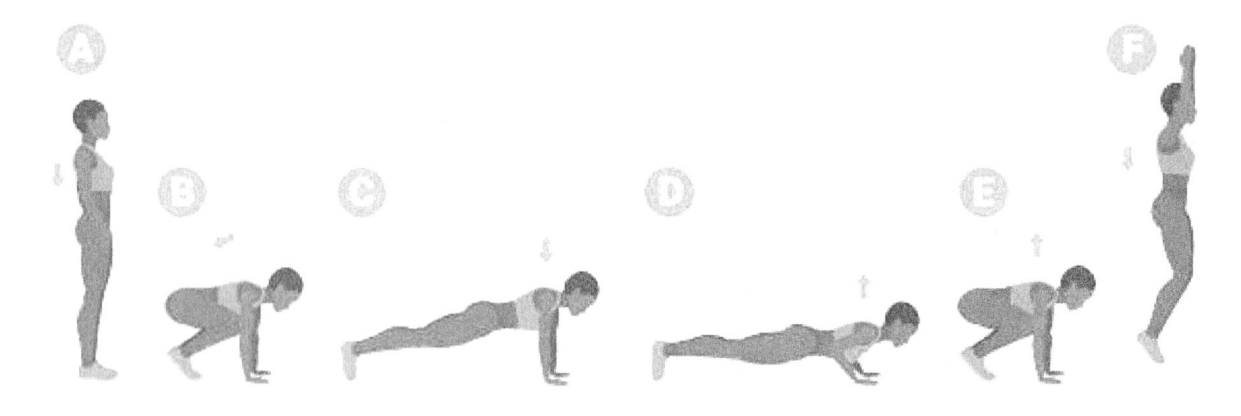

How effective are burpees?

Fortunately all that work is totally worth the effort. The burpee works your arms, back, chest, center, glutes and legs - and so on, it works it. What's more, burpees likewise spike your pulse as much as running for a transport does - one explanation it's a firm #1 among the intense cardio exercise swarm.

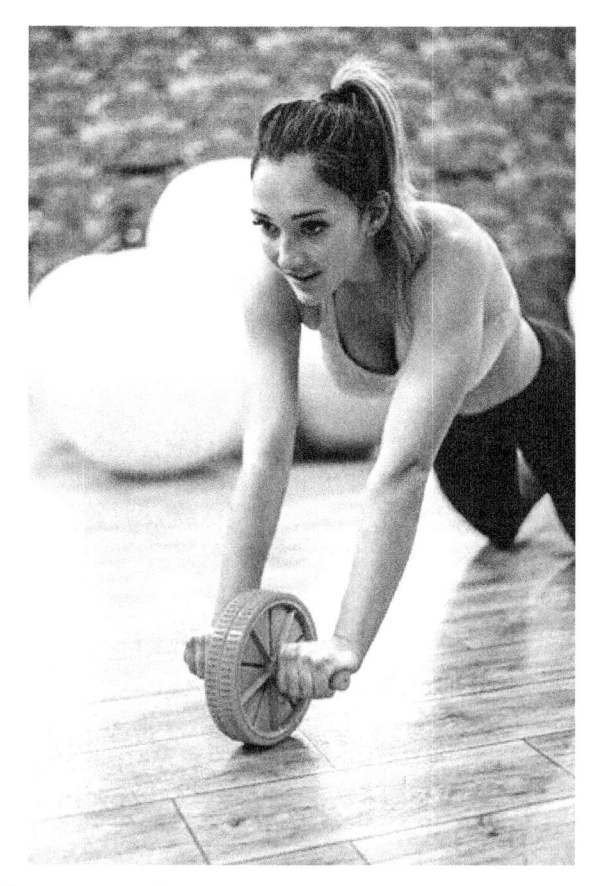

How effective are ab rollouts?

The rolling out development basically works your lats and deltoids, though the last part of the development — the moving in segment — truly focuses on your center, explicitly your rectus abdominis.

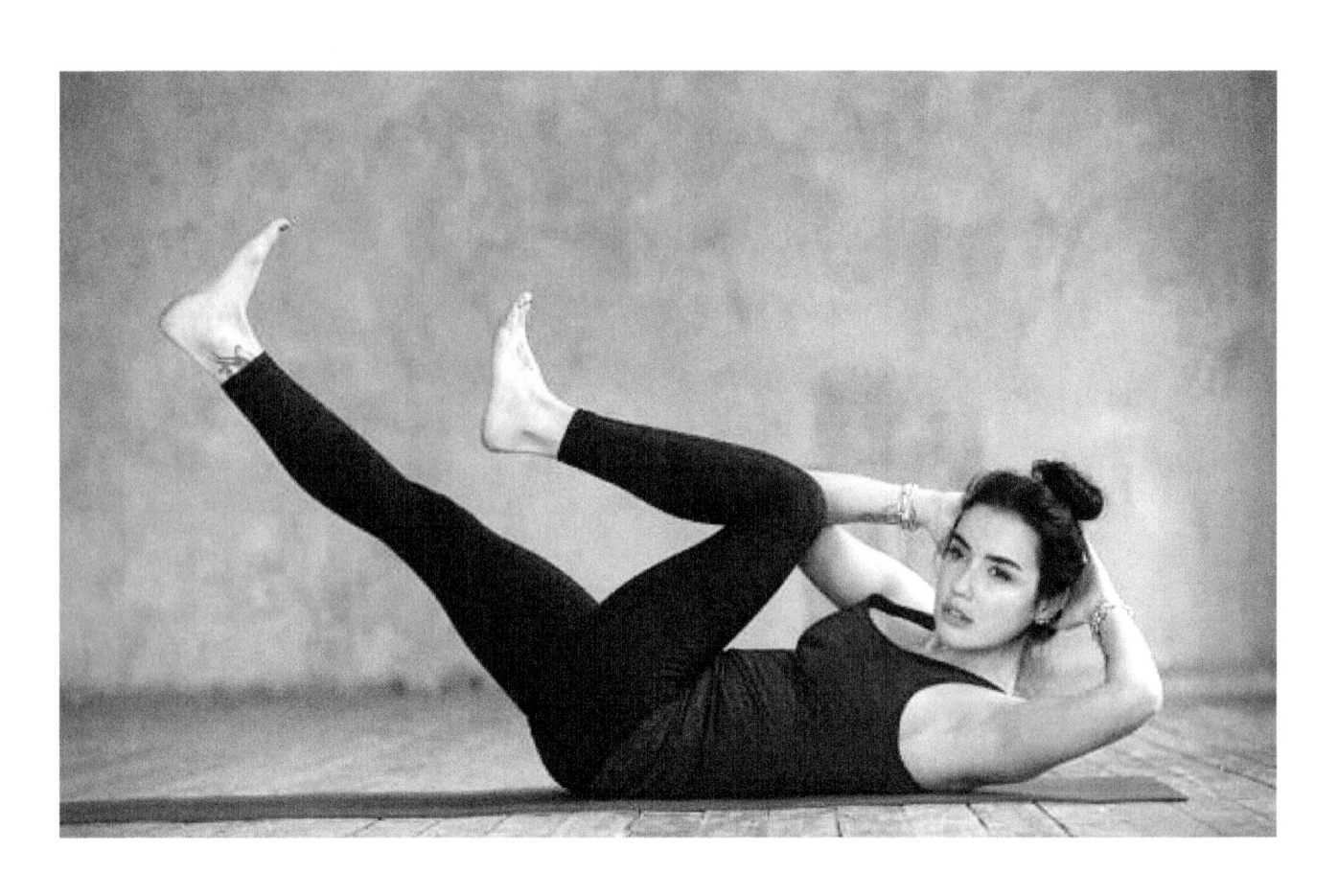

How effective are oblique crunches?

The slanted crunch completely connects with the stomach wall and the obliques and assists with chiseling the midsection. This exercise reinforces the back, fixes the center, conditions the abs, and further develops equilibrium and adaptability.

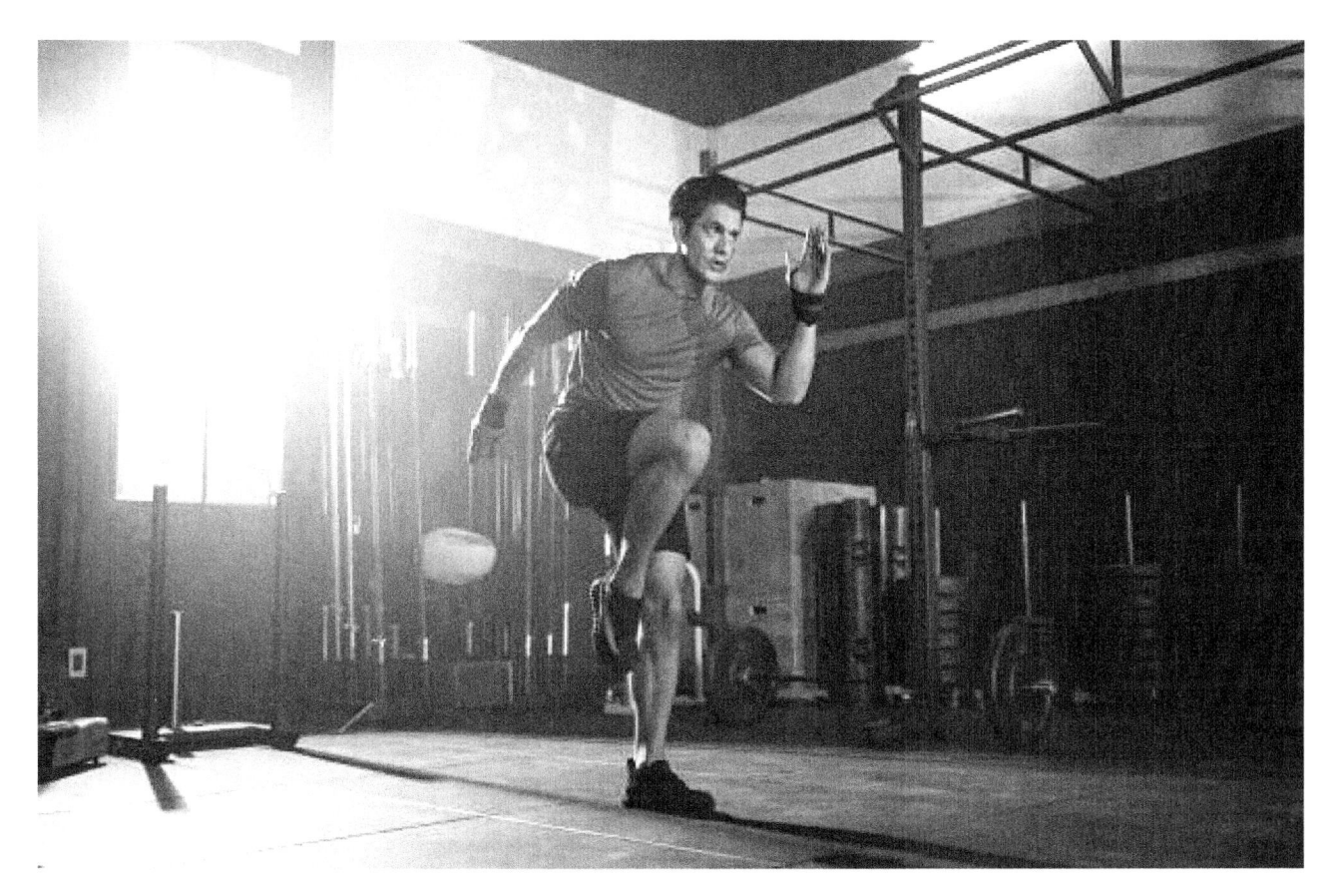

How effective are high knees?

High knees enact your quadriceps, hamstrings, calves, glutes, and hip flexors, working on solid perseverance, equilibrium, and coordination in these muscles. When done at a focused energy and with bouncing or unstable knee drives, they can likewise further develop power in your lower body.

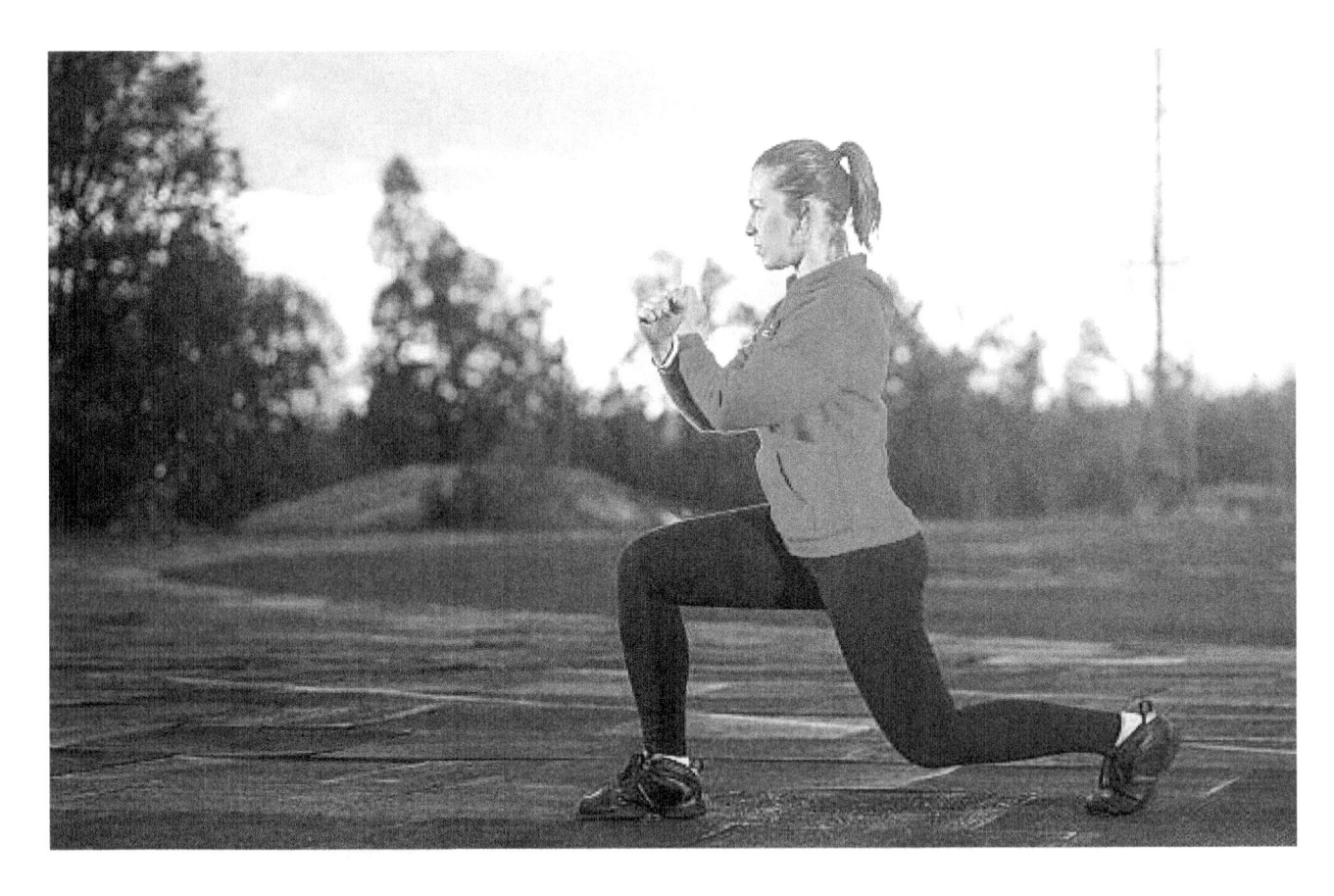

How effective are split squats?

The split squat is one of the best activities for preparing the lower body, and when done accurately, works the majority of the muscles in the lower body. One more advantage of the split squat is that it is a solitary leg work out, which can be utilized to address irregular characteristics from left to right.

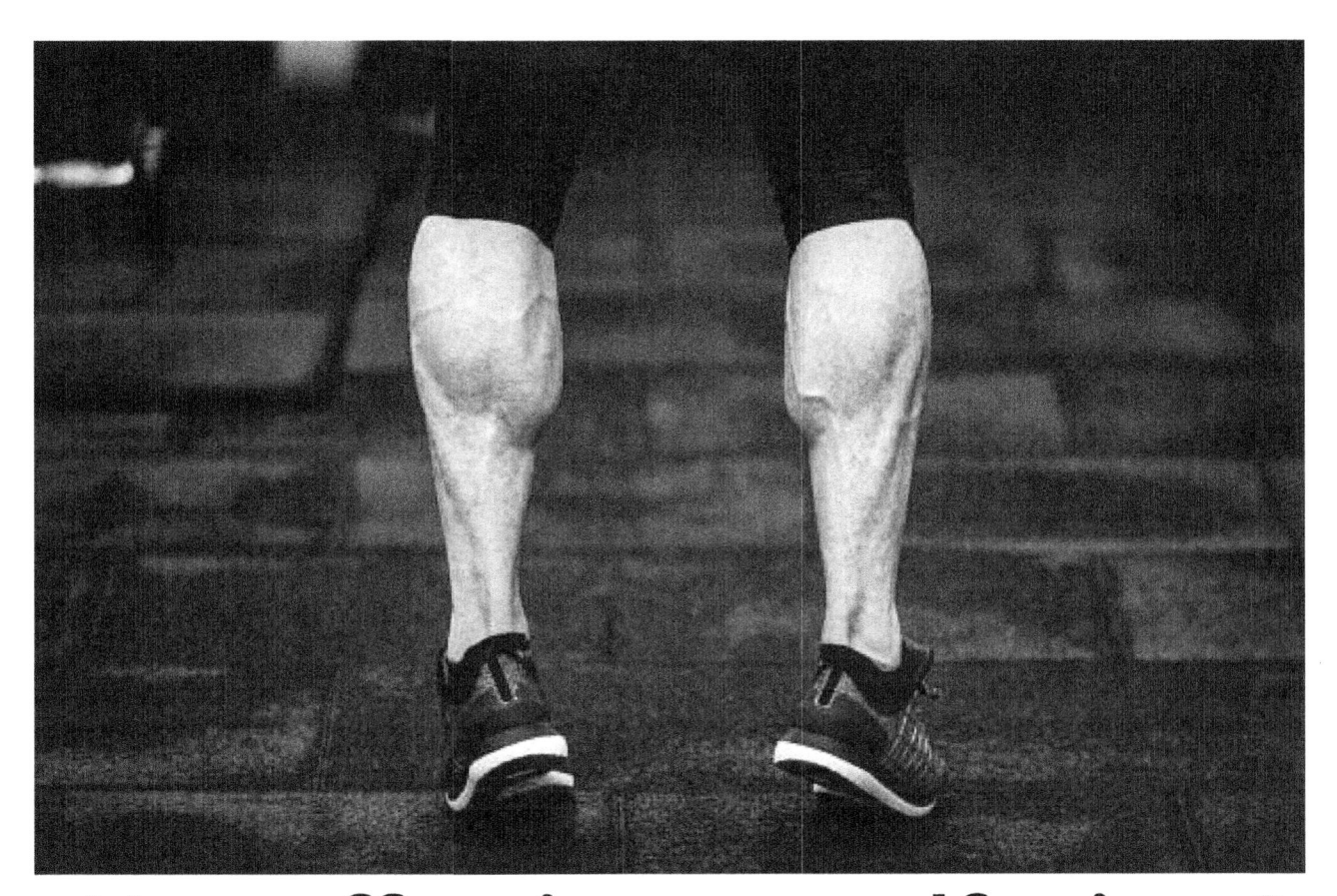

How effective are calf raises?

It's great for improving ankle stability and overall balance. Calf raises are also excellent for stretching the plantar muscles of the foot and making it more supple." Beyond the calf muscles, the benefits of calf raises carry over to other parts of your leg.

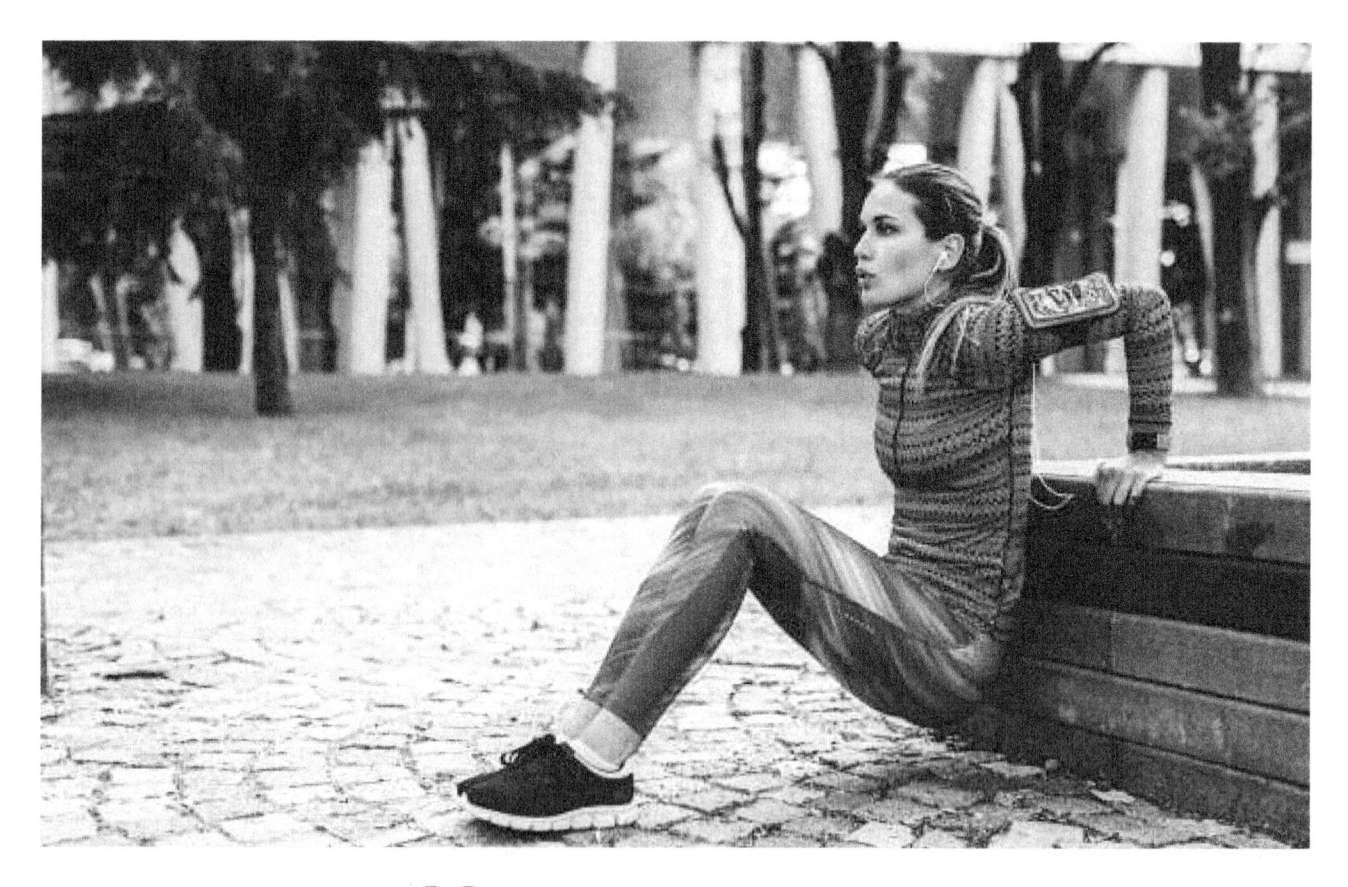

How effective are dips?

Dips are viewed as a chest area squeezing exercise that principally construct greater and more grounded rear arm muscles, however they likewise hit the chest, shoulders and, surprisingly, the back. Truth be told, Plunges are one of the most outstanding activities for creating in general chest area strength and size.

LATERAL TOE TAPS

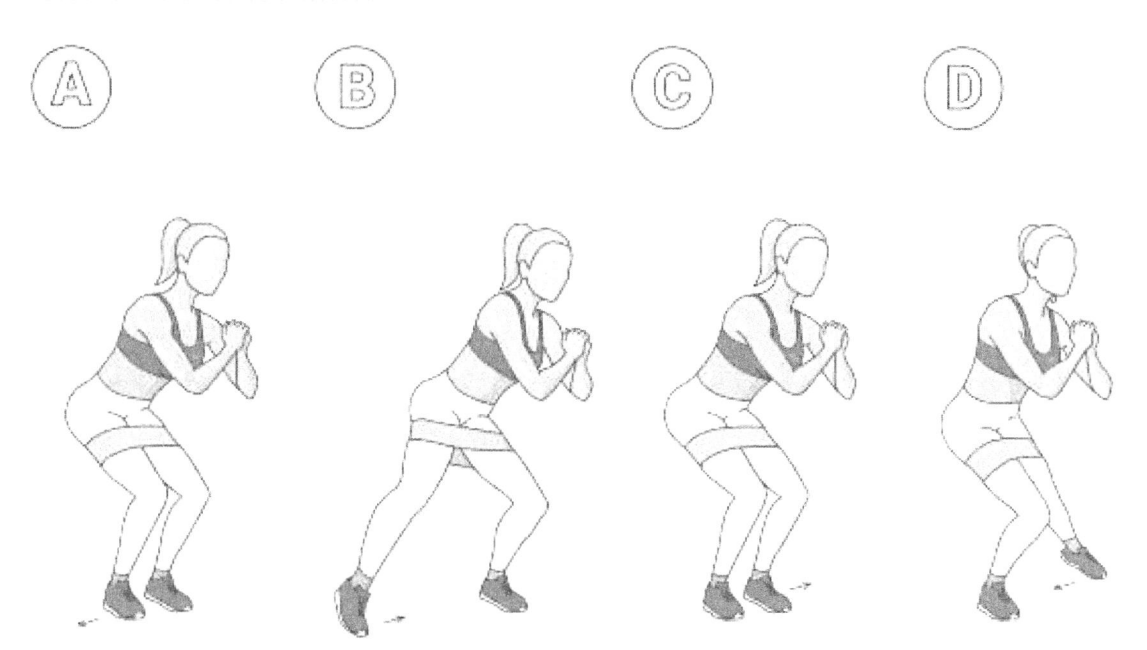

Ⓐ　　　Ⓑ　　　Ⓒ　　　Ⓓ

How effective are toe taps?

This rendition of the activity is perfect for raising your pulse, focusing on the muscles in your lower body, consuming calories, and further developing velocity, equilibrium, and foot-dealing with abilities. You depend on serious areas of strength for the in your glutes, hip flexors, quads, hamstrings, calves, and center to appropriately play out a standing toe tap.

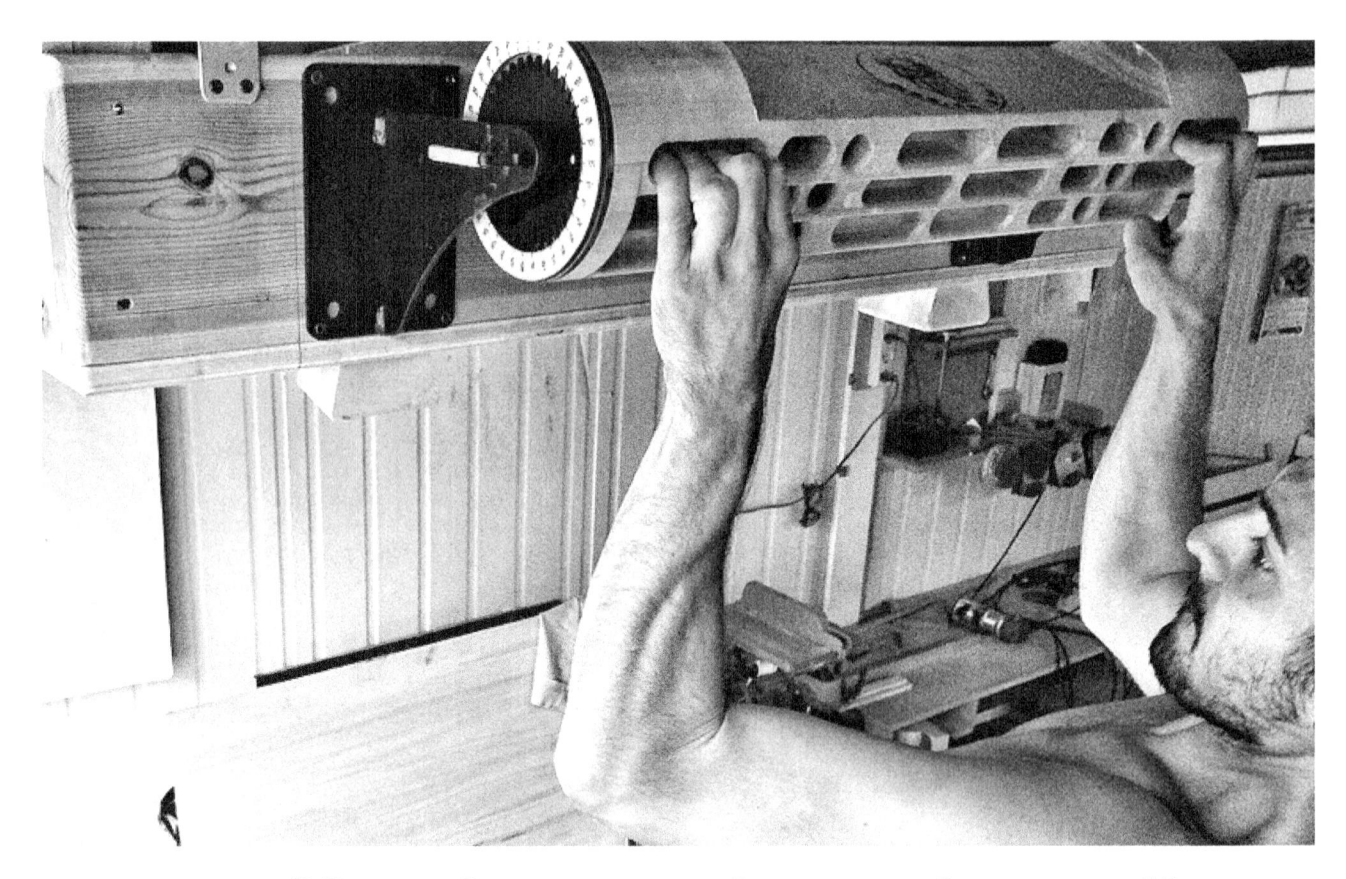

How effective are hang boarding?

There is no doubt that hangboarding is one of the most outstanding ways of expanding grasp strength and chest area power. On the off chance that you're not a hereditary victory worked for climbing, arriving at your full climbing potential is possible important.

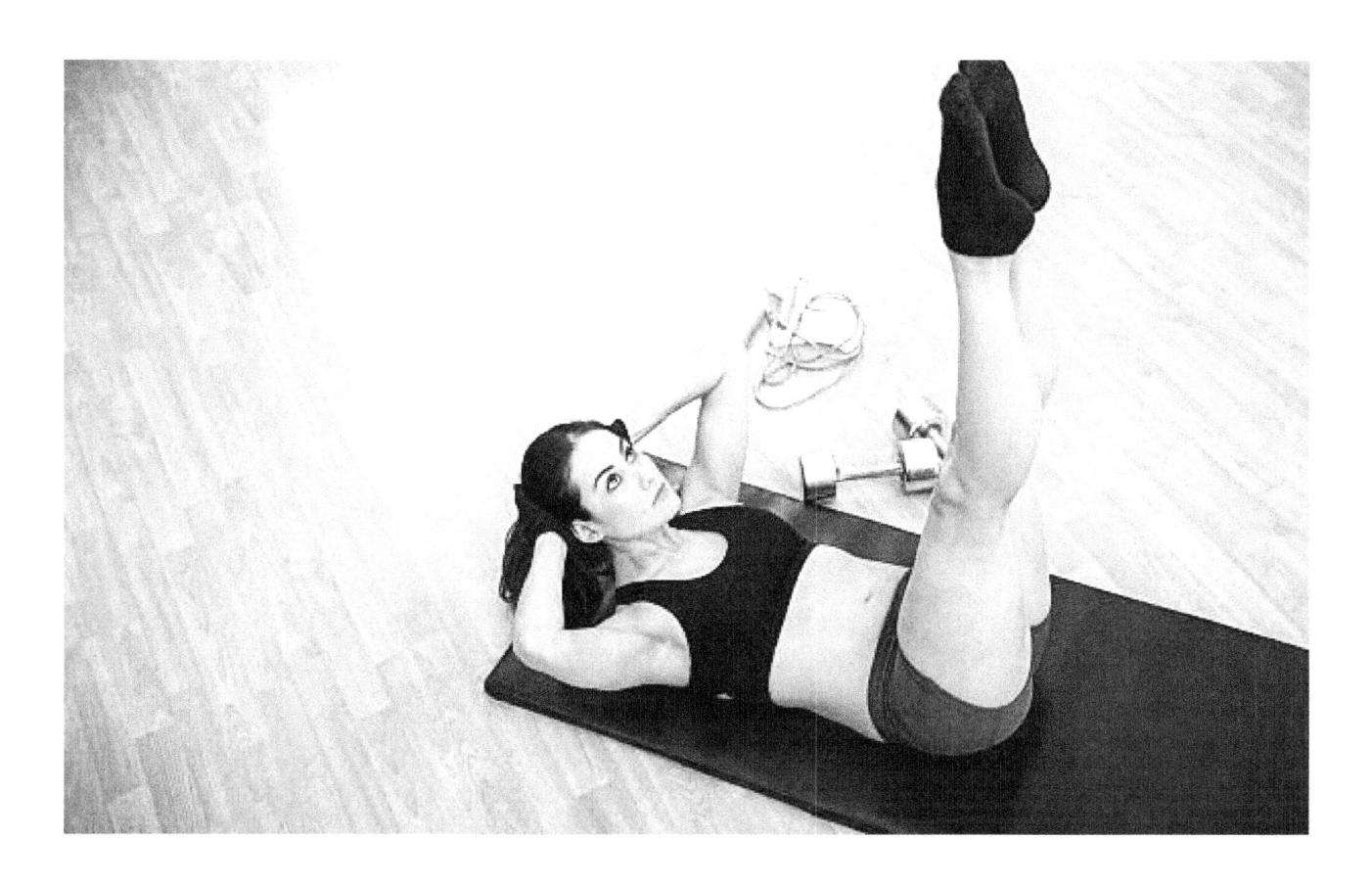

How effective are leg lifts?

Leg lifts work your center for better adjustment and equilibrium, which prompts better generally speaking control of your body. Leg lifts work the lower abs, however they additionally work the internal thighs (which in Pilates, are viewed as a feature of the center). Concentrates on show that having a steady center is fundamental in forestalling injury.

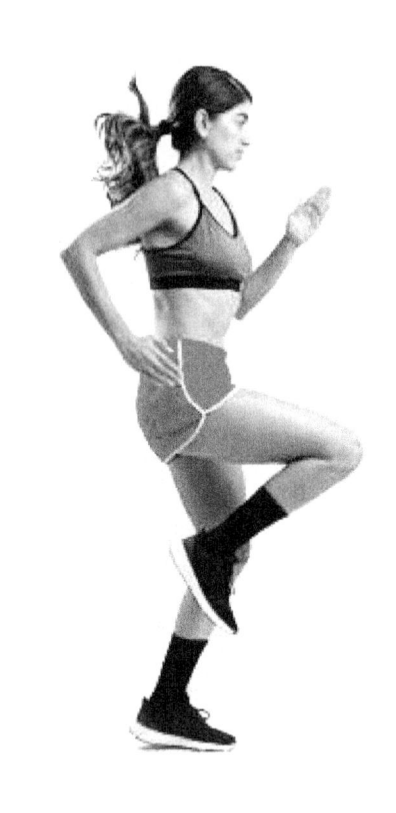

How effective is running in place?

Running in place raises your pulse, further develops glucose levels, and consumes calories and fat, all of which assist with weight reduction. You'll likewise support cardiovascular capability, upgrade lung limit, and further develop dissemination.

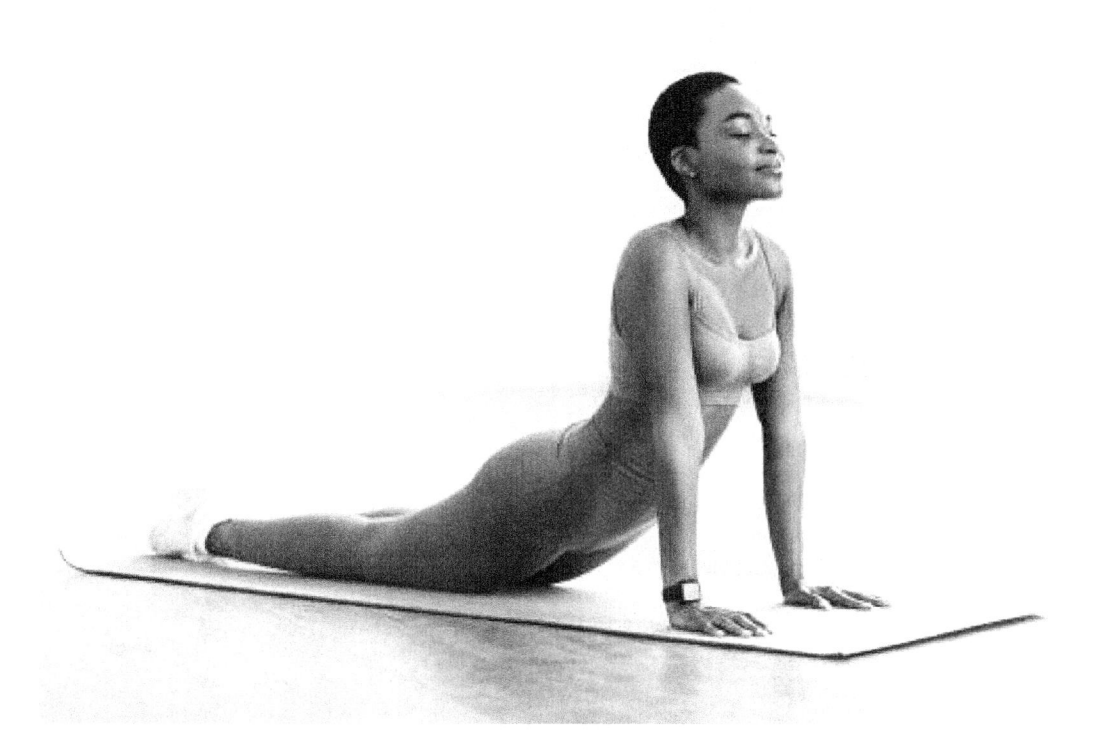

How effective is Yoga?

Yoga further develops strength, equilibrium and adaptability. Sluggish developments and profound breathing increment blood stream and warm up muscles, while holding a posture can develop fortitude. Balance on one foot, while holding the other foot to your calf or over the knee (however never on the knee) at a right point.

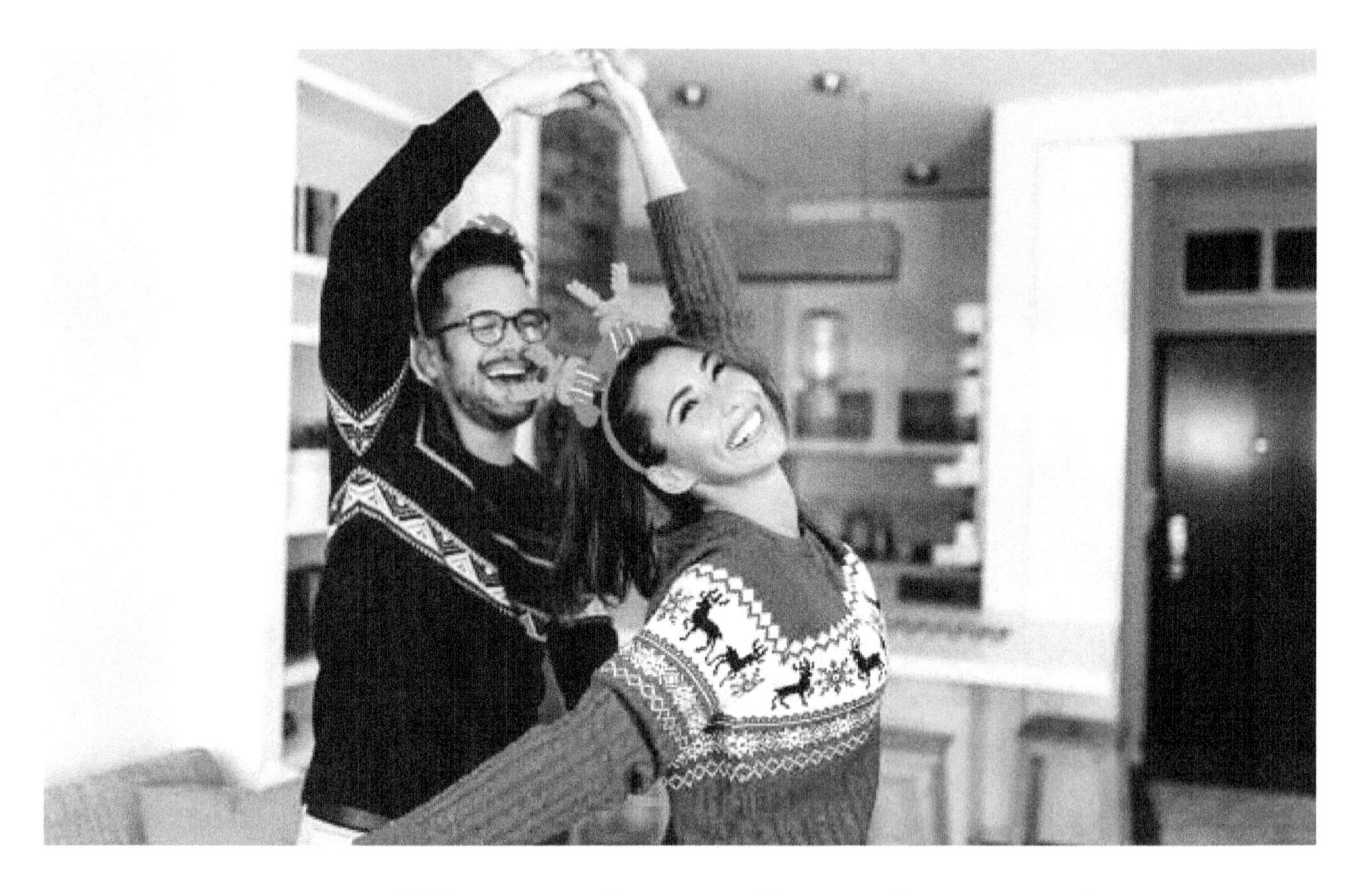

How effective is dancing?

Dancing is an entire body exercise that is really fun. It's great for your heart, it makes you more grounded, and it can assist with equilibrium and coordination. A 30-minute dance class consumes somewhere in the range of 130 and 250 calories, about equivalent to running.

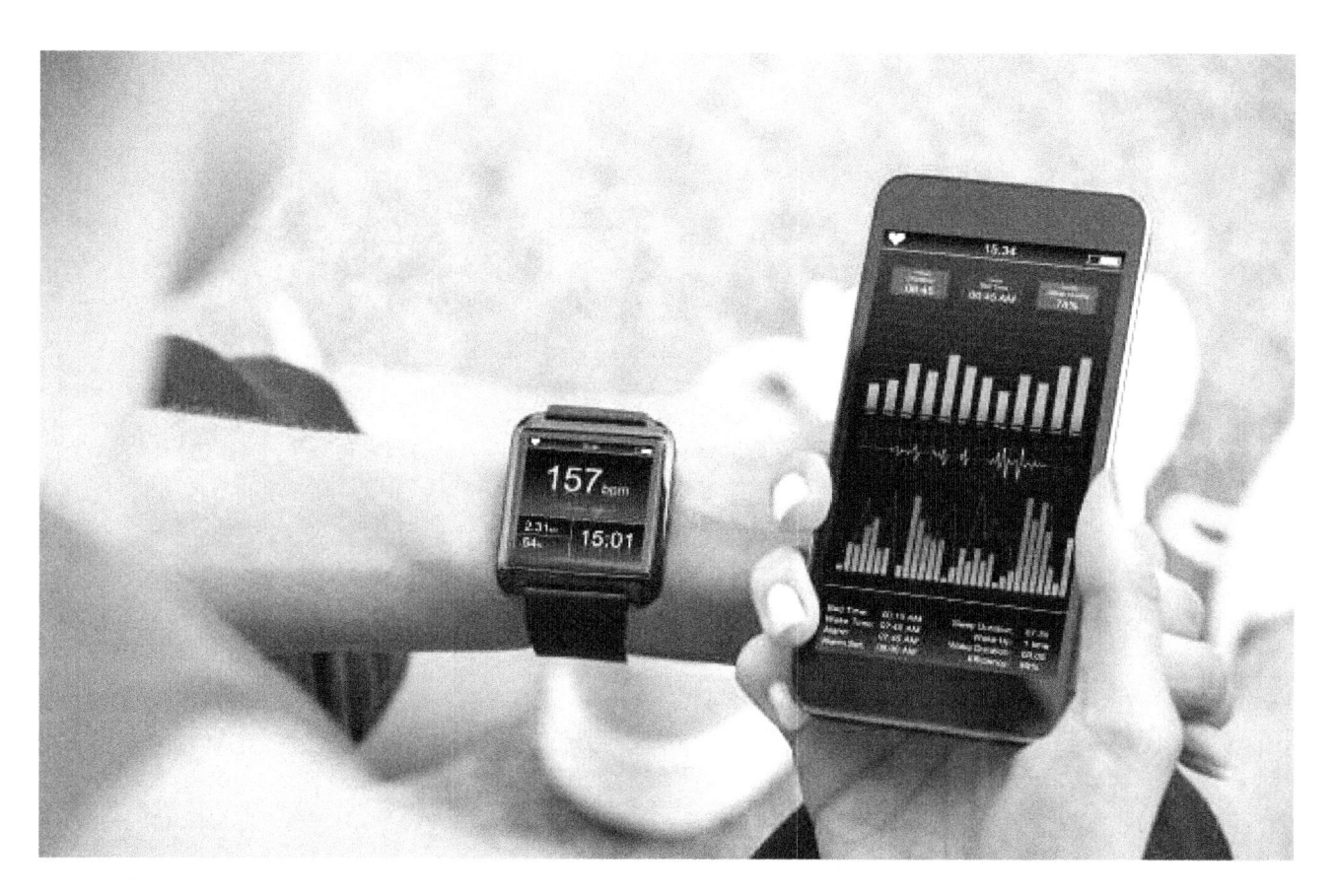

How effective are workout apps?

Other examination proposes that wellness applications certainly work, yet are particularly successful when they're customized to the client. At the point when highlights incorporate things like preparation objectives, specific weight control plans or contact with "genuine live coaches," individuals are more spurred to reliably resolve more.

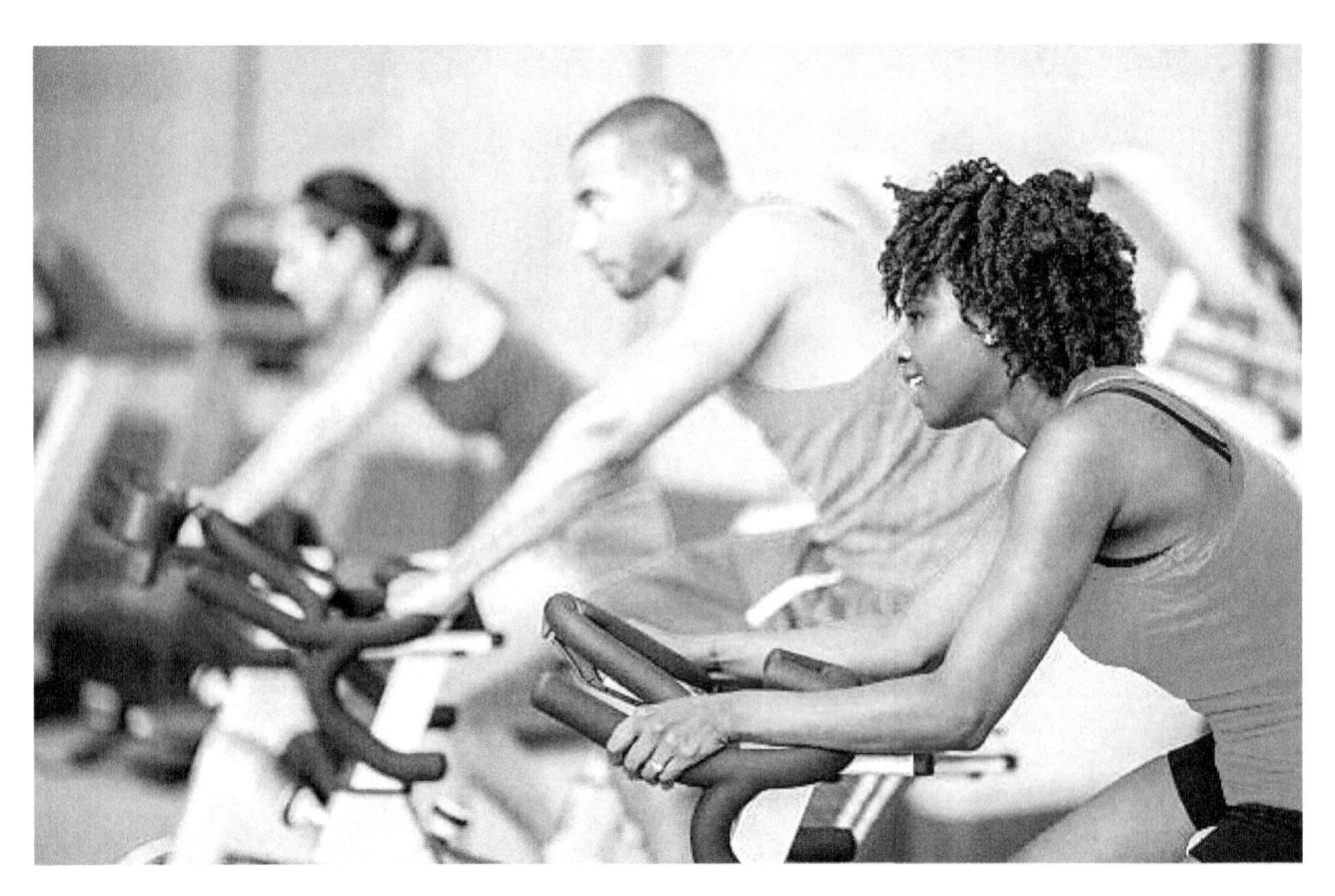

How effective are spin bikes?

Riding a fixed activity bicycle is a productive and successful method for consuming calories and muscle to fat ratio while reinforcing your heart, lungs, and muscles. Contrasted with a few different sorts of cardio hardware, an exercise bike puts less weight on your joints, however it actually gives a great high-impact exercise.

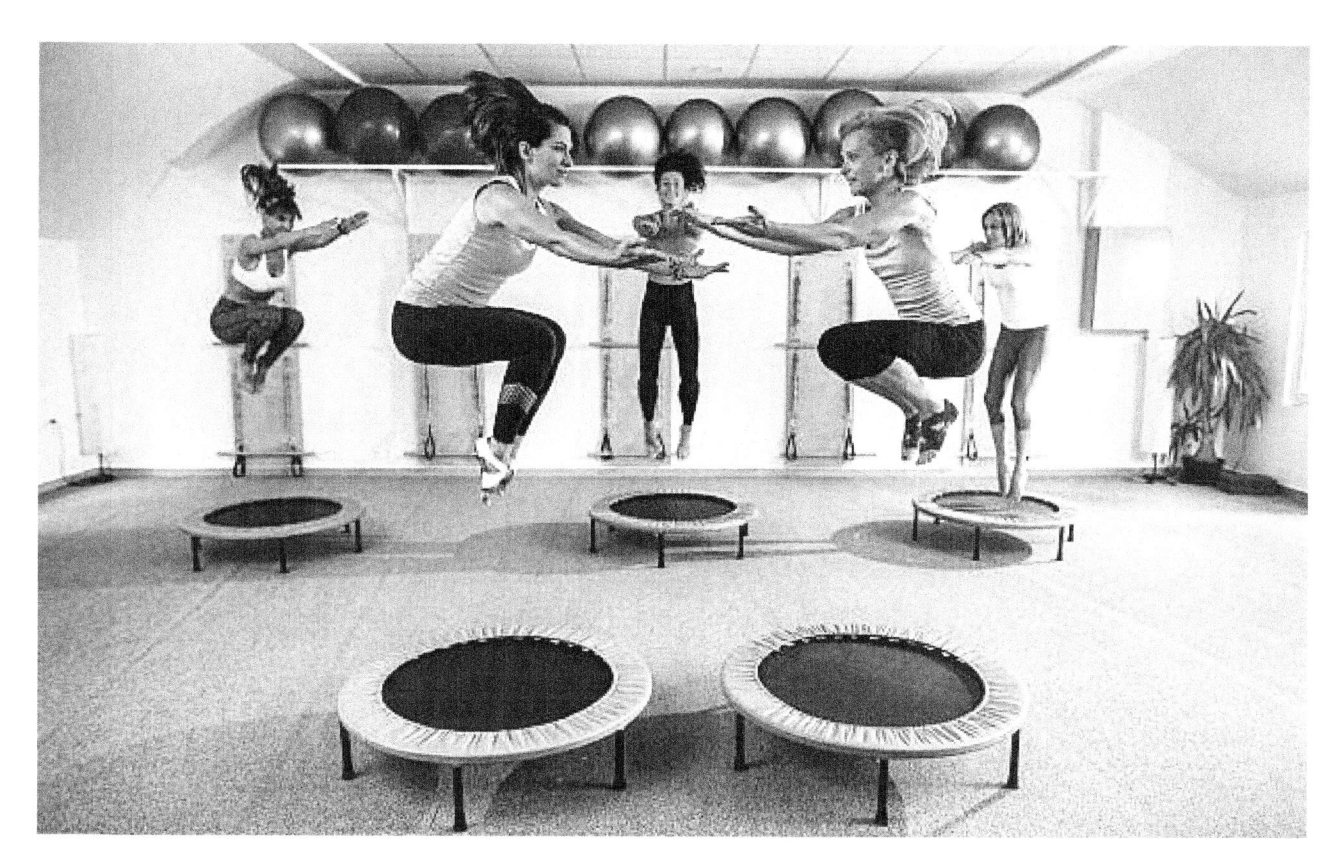

How effective is trampoline jumping?

They can assist you with growing better equilibrium, coordination, and coordinated abilities. These activities focus on your back, center, and leg muscles. You'll likewise work your arms, neck, and glutes. Research shows that bouncing decidedly affects bone well-being, and it might assist with working on bone thickness and strength.

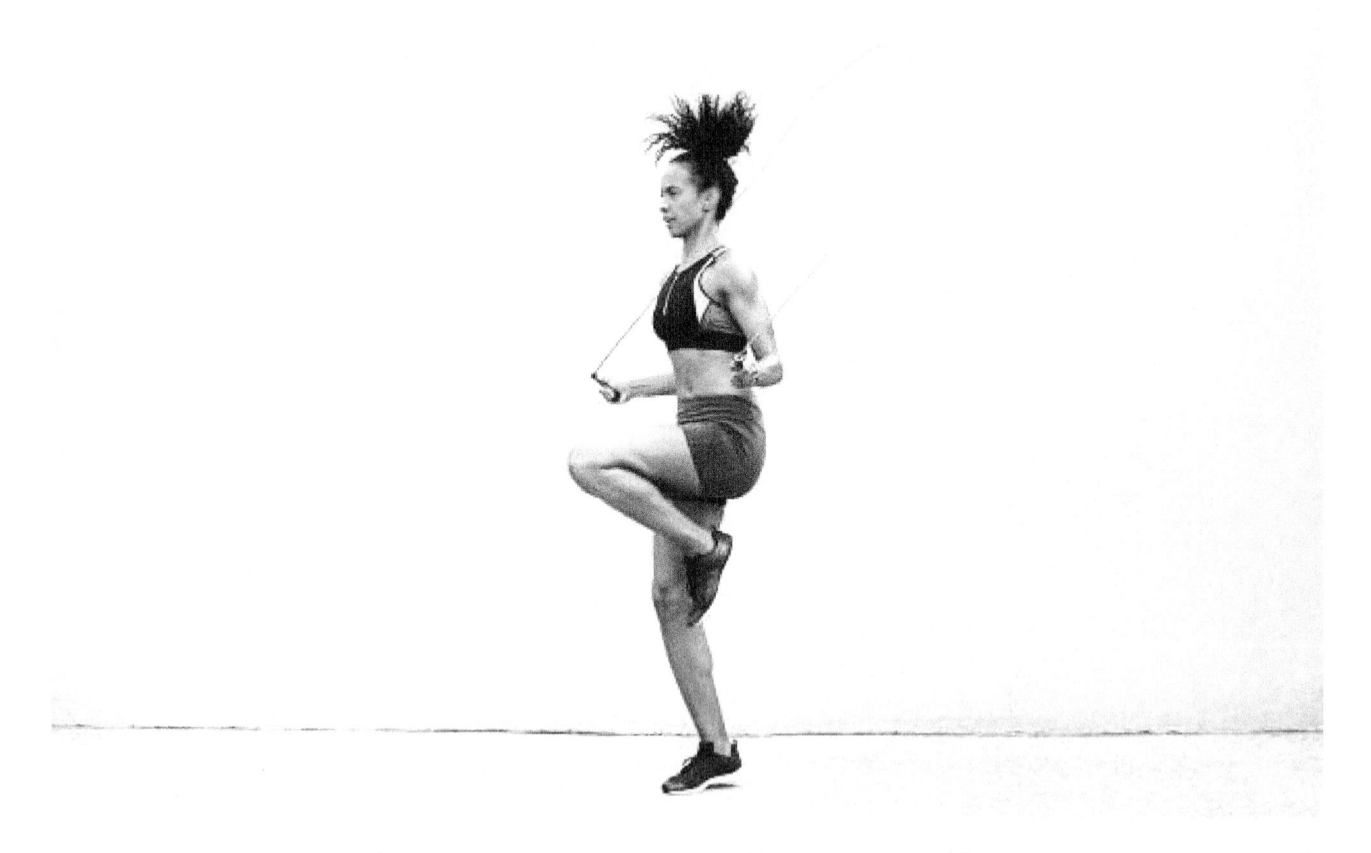

How effective is jumping rope?

Working out with a rope is a successful exercise that can consume numerous calories in a brief period of time. For instance, 20 minutes of bounce rope can wreck to 241 calories for a 200-pound (91-kg) individual.

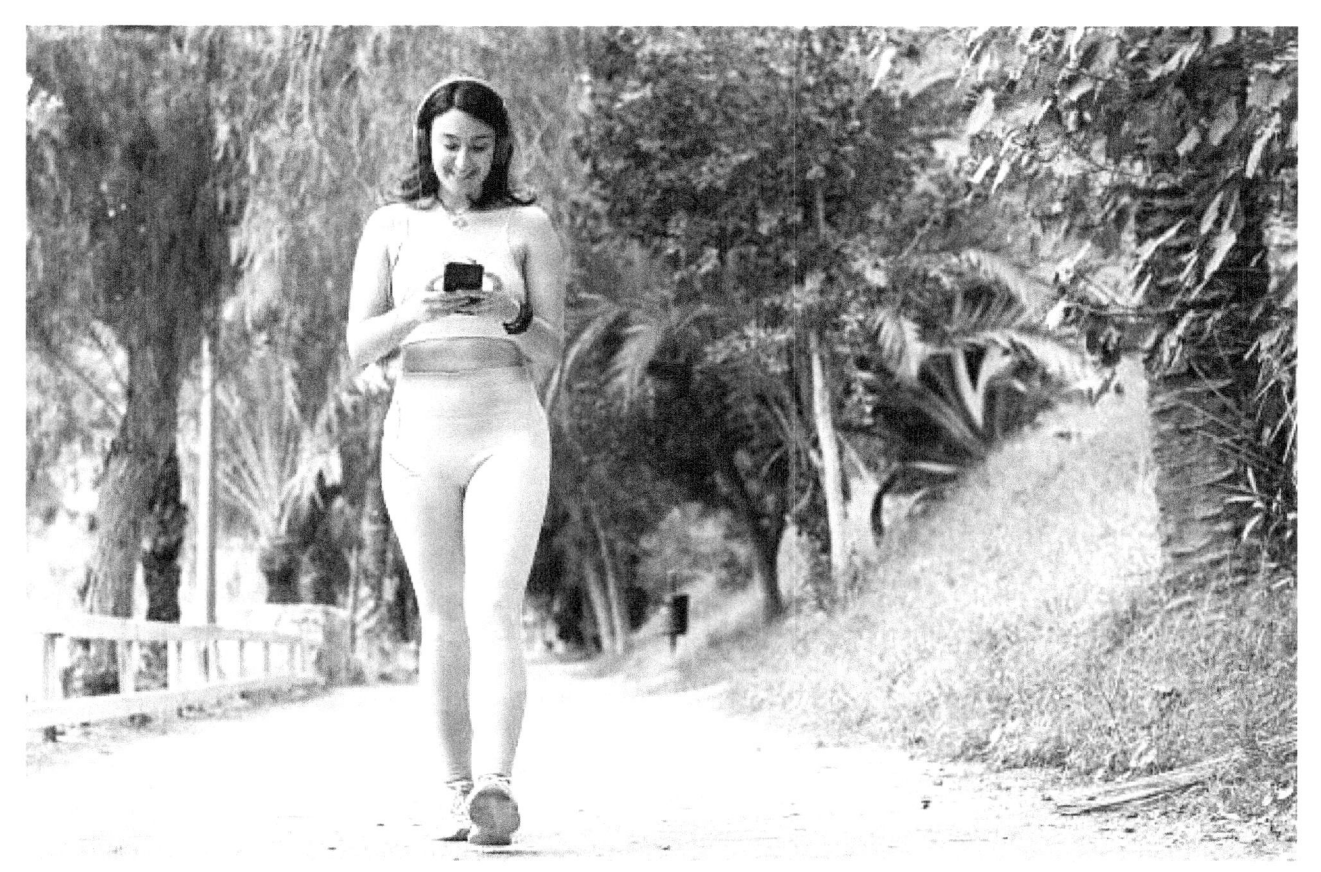

How effective is walking?

Walking is a kind of cardiovascular actual work, which builds your pulse. This further develops blood stream and can bring down pulse. It assists with helping energy levels by delivering specific chemicals like endorphins and conveying oxygen all through the body.

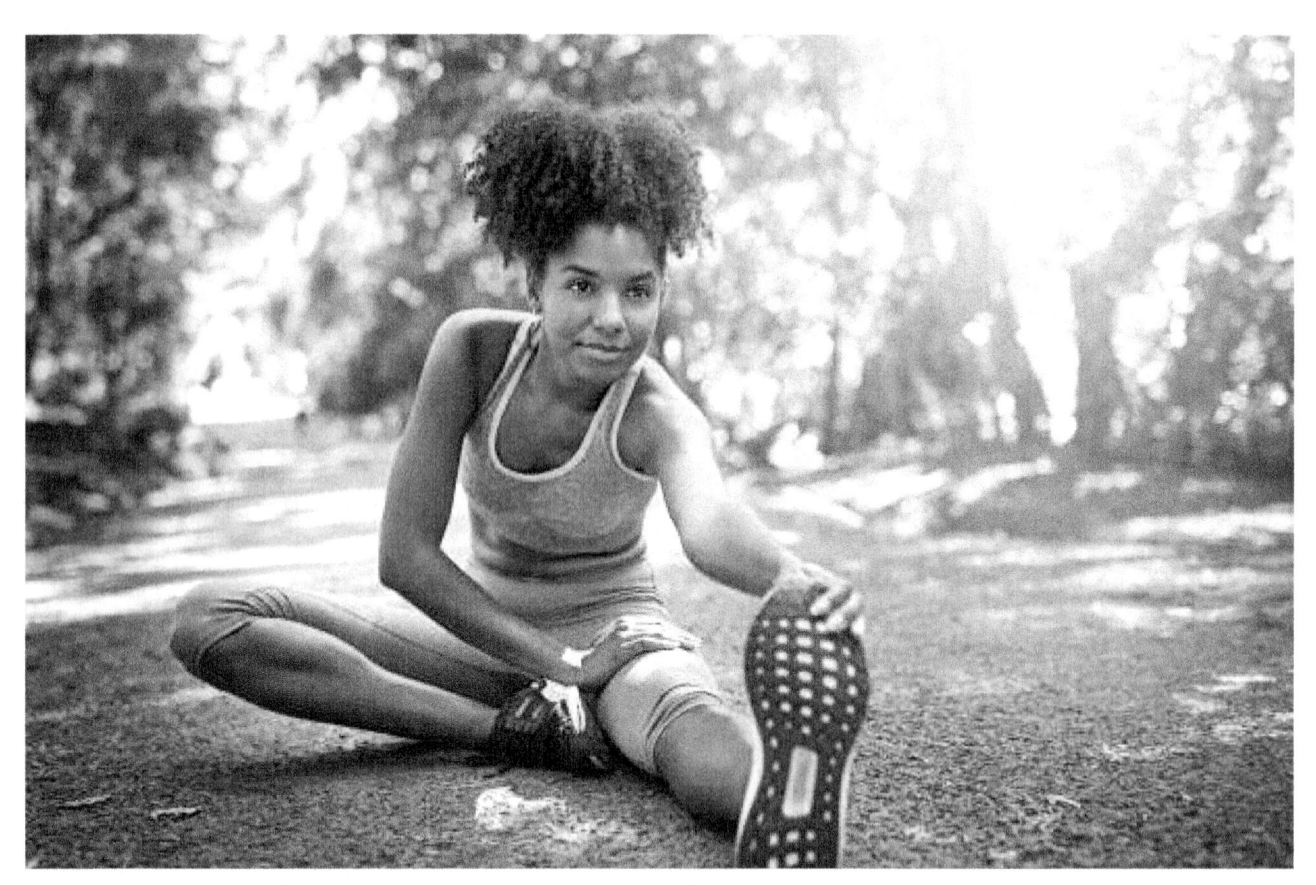

How effective is stretching?

Stretching keeps the muscles flexible, strong, and healthy, and we need that flexibility to maintain a range of motion in the joints. Without it, the muscles shorten and become tight. Then, when you call on the muscles for activity, they are weak and unable to extend all the way.

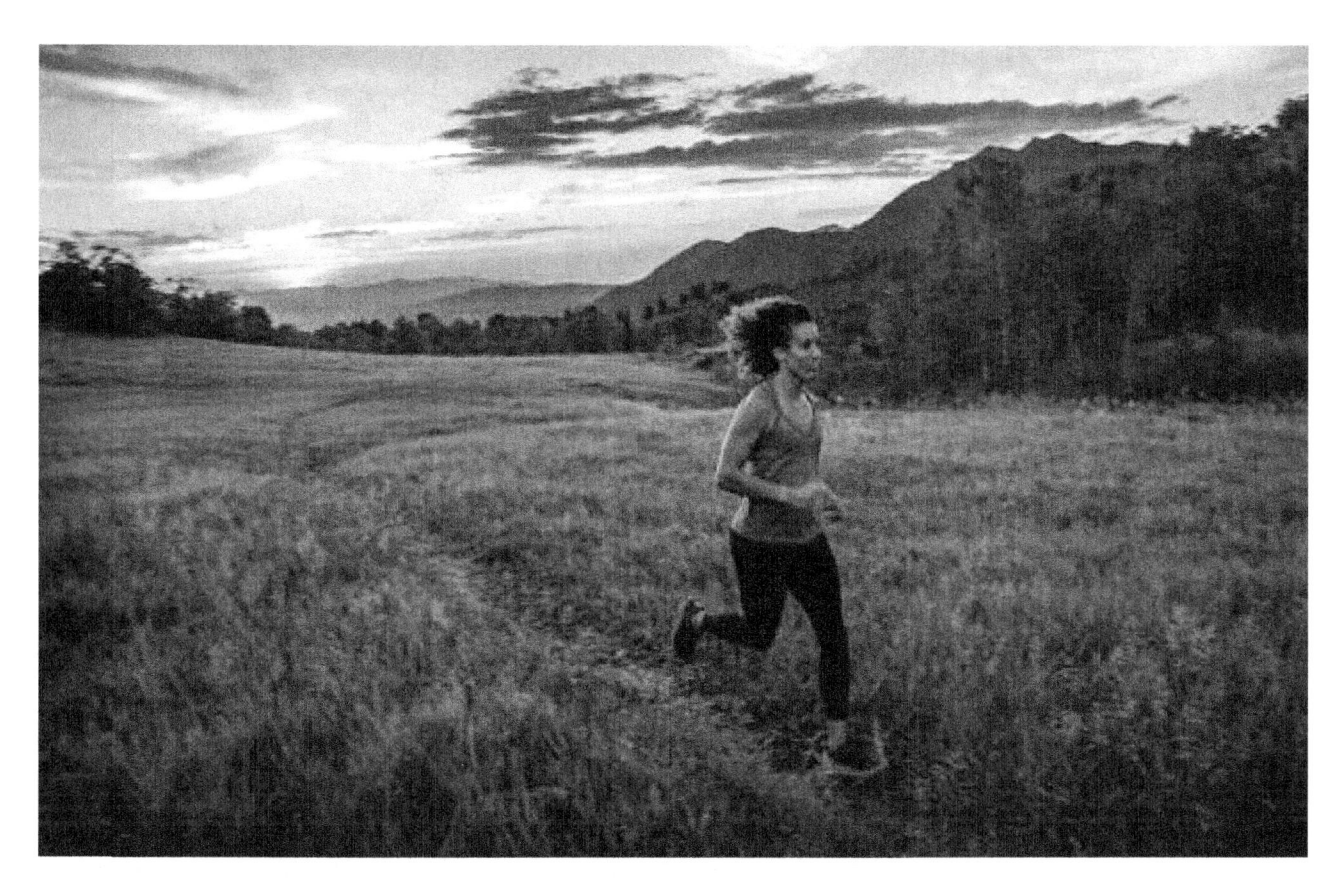

How effective is jogging?

Running is a successful movement to consume calories both during the activity and after its consummation. As a matter of fact, running wears out a significant number of calories when contrasted with some other type of cardio exercise.

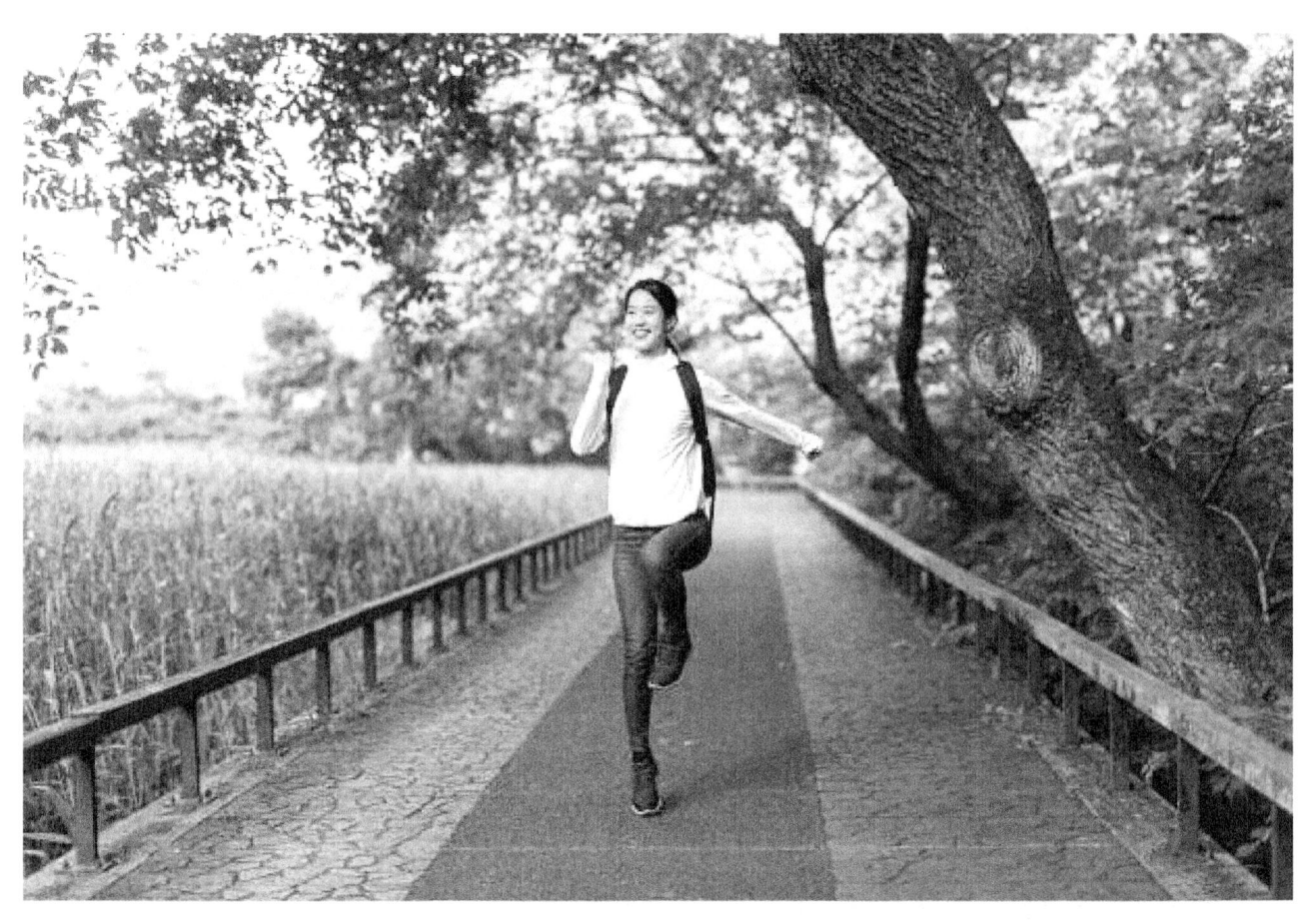

How effective is skipping?

It further develops coordination and coordinated movements

Skipping includes coordination to time your leap with the rope. Research has shown that it further develops coordination, equilibrium and essential development abilities in kids. These are significant wellness parts for further down the road as they lessen our possibilities of outings and falls.

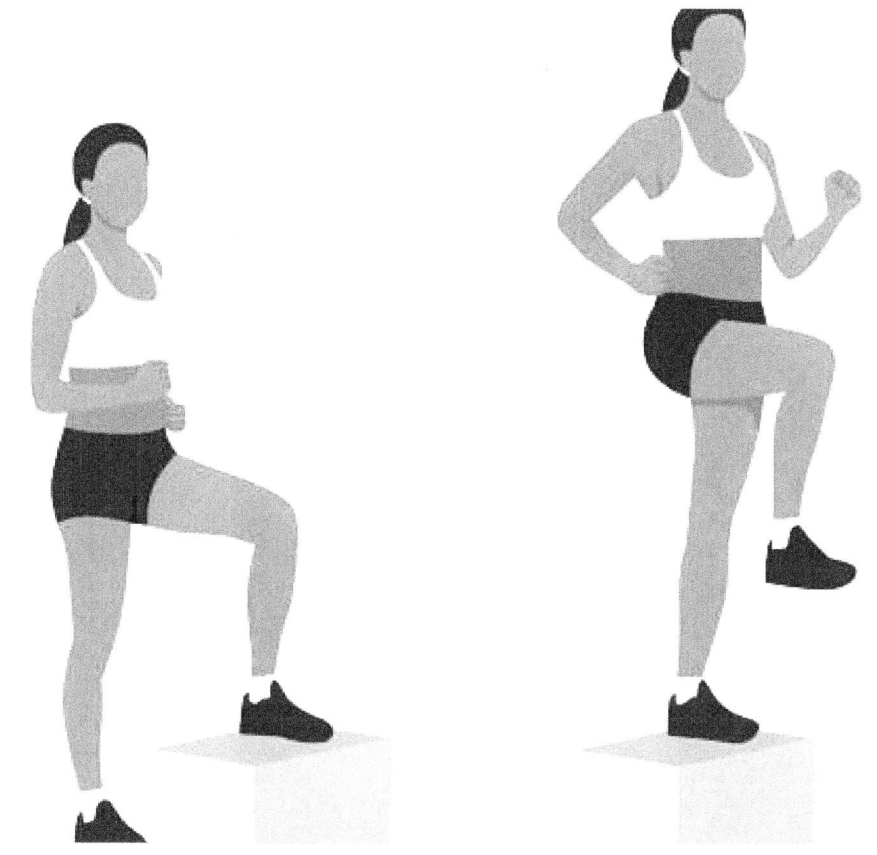

How effective are step-ups?

4 Advantages of Doing Step aerobics
Step-ups can increment leg strength. Step-ups initiate muscle bunches all through your lower body, including your quadriceps, hamstrings, glutes, and adductors.
Step-ups might out strength uneven characters. ...
Step-ups can upgrade adjustment. ...
Step-ups are adaptable.

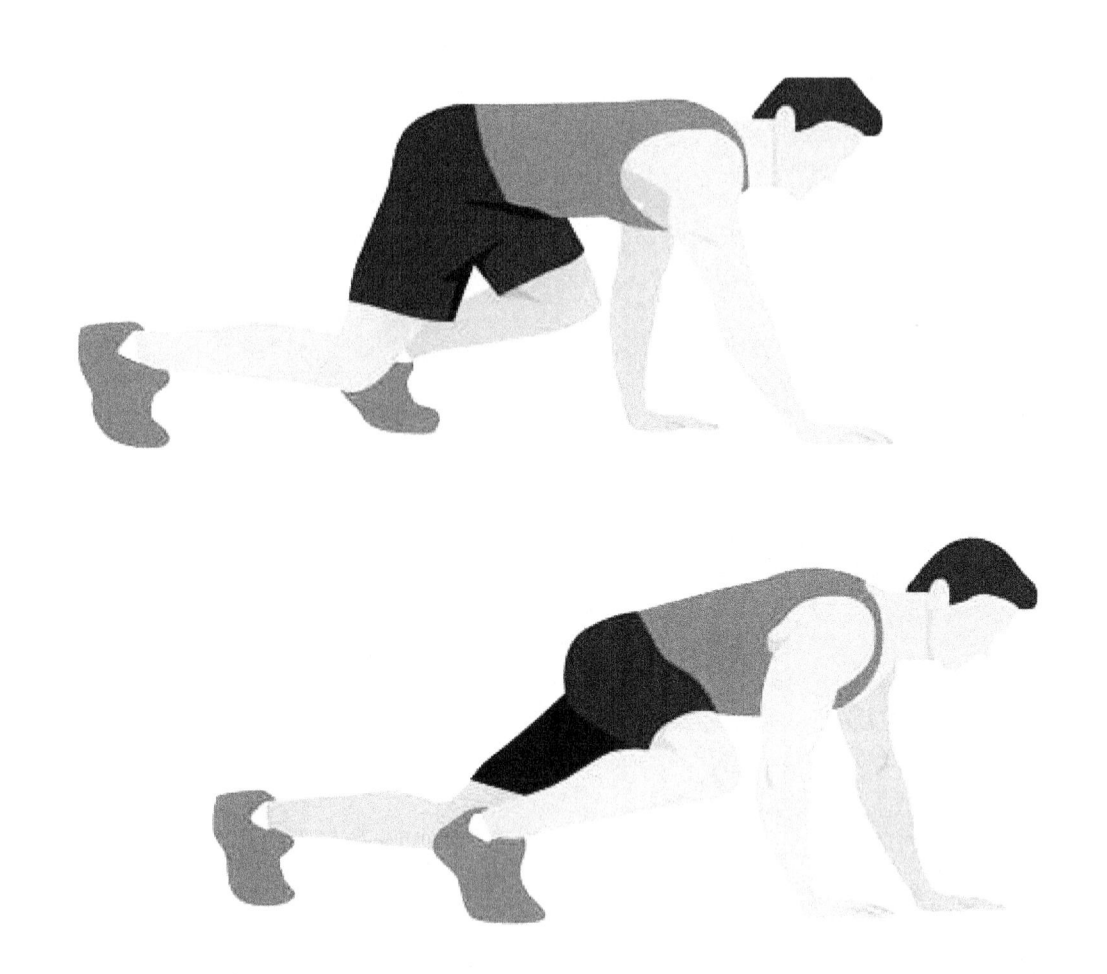

How effective is bear crawling?

While playing out the bear crawl, you utilize pretty much every muscle in the body. This exercise works the shoulders (deltoids), chest and back, glutes, quadriceps, hamstrings, and center. Do bear crawls routinely and you can develop all out body fortitude and perseverance.

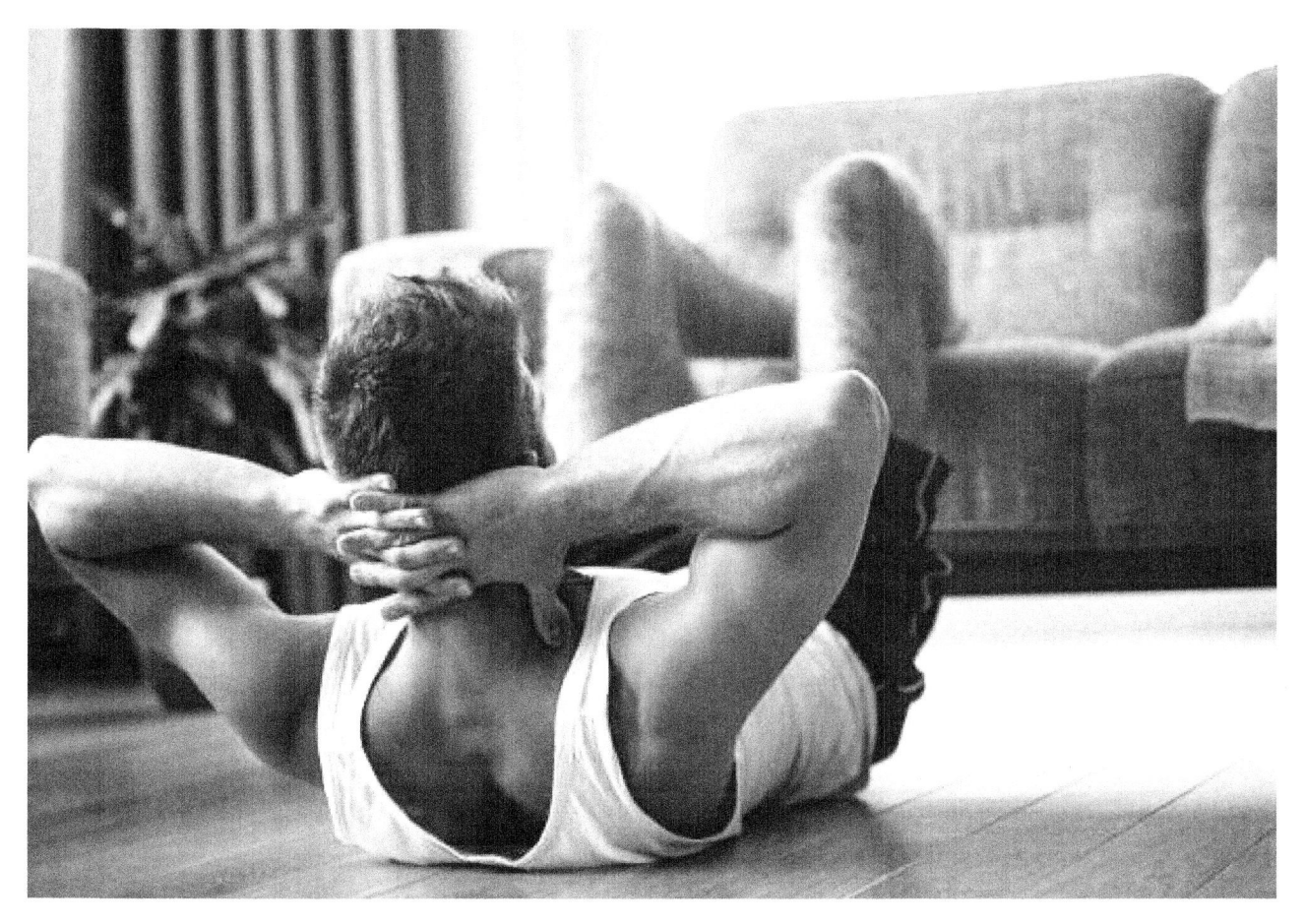

How effective are crunches?

Like situps, crunches assist you with building muscle. In any case, not at all like situps, they work just the stomach muscles. This extraordinary muscle detachment makes them a famous activity for individuals attempting to get super strong abs. This likewise makes them ideal for reinforcing your center, which incorporates your lower back muscles and obliques.

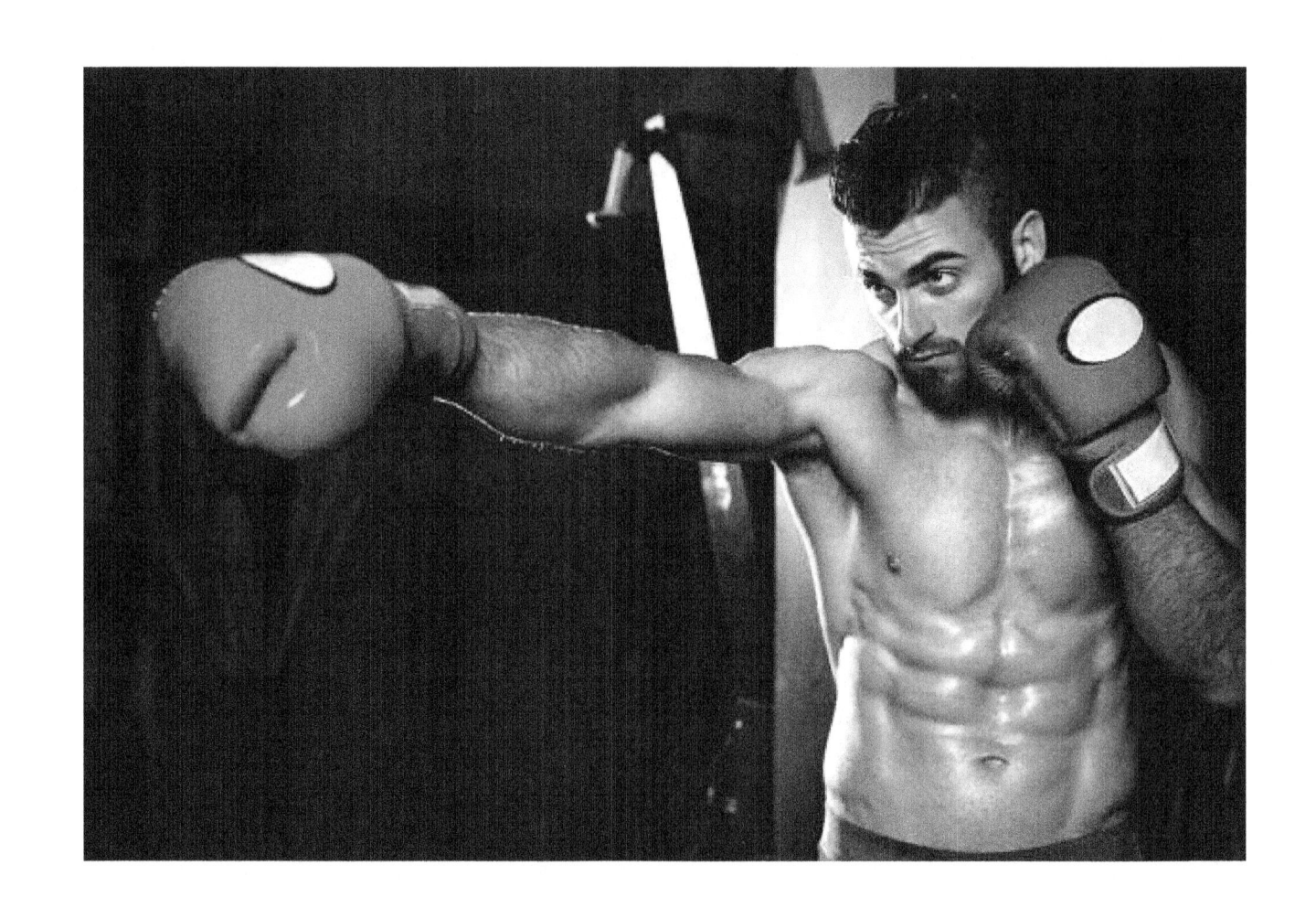

How effective is shadowboxing?

Shadowboxing is an incredible full-body exercise that tones muscles, takes out pressure, and increase your boxing match-up. Additionally, you don't require gear!

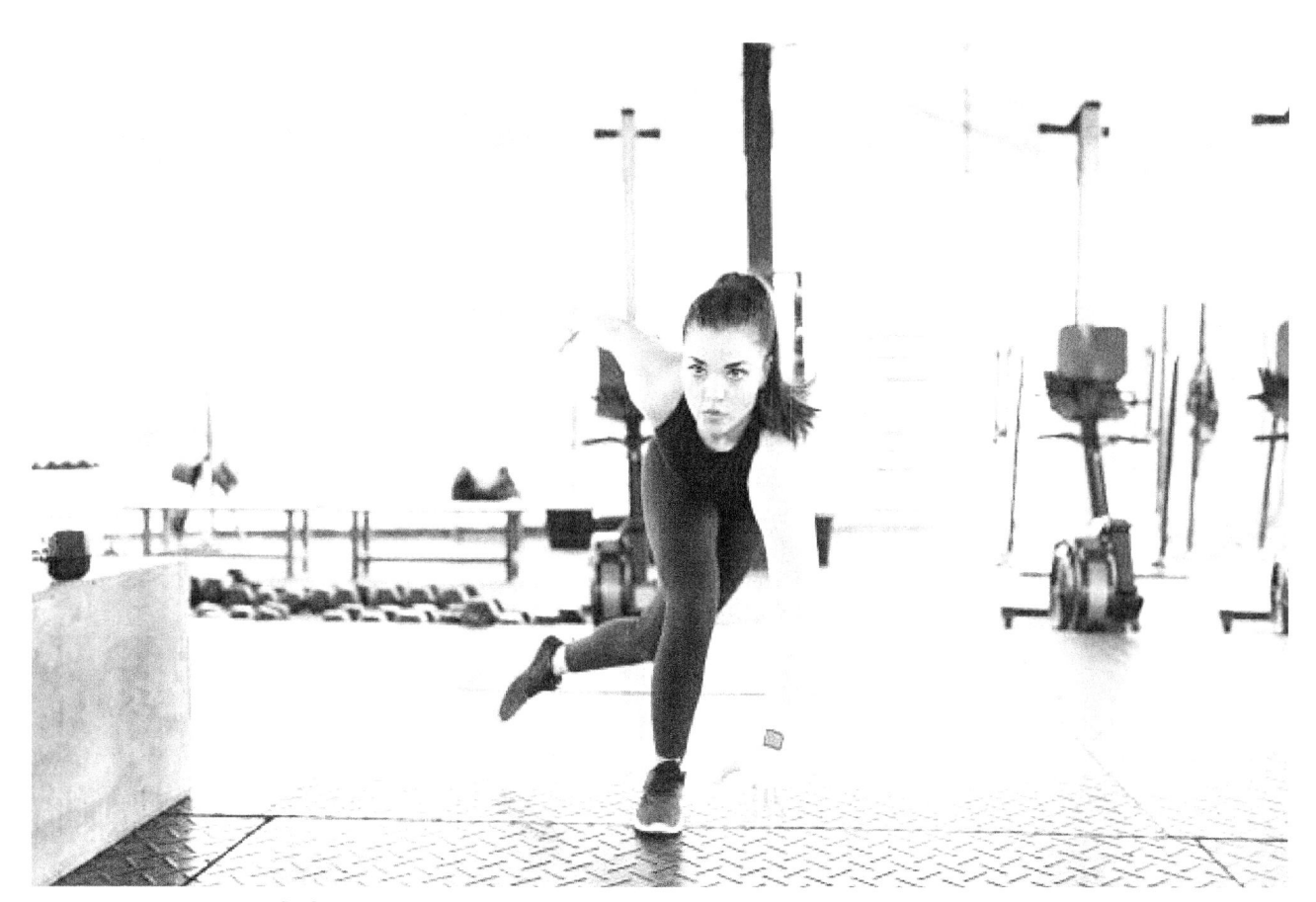

How effective are lateral bounds?

The lateral bound assists train with driving creation. It is critical that the competitor can keep up with control of the hips, knees and lower legs during unstable developments.

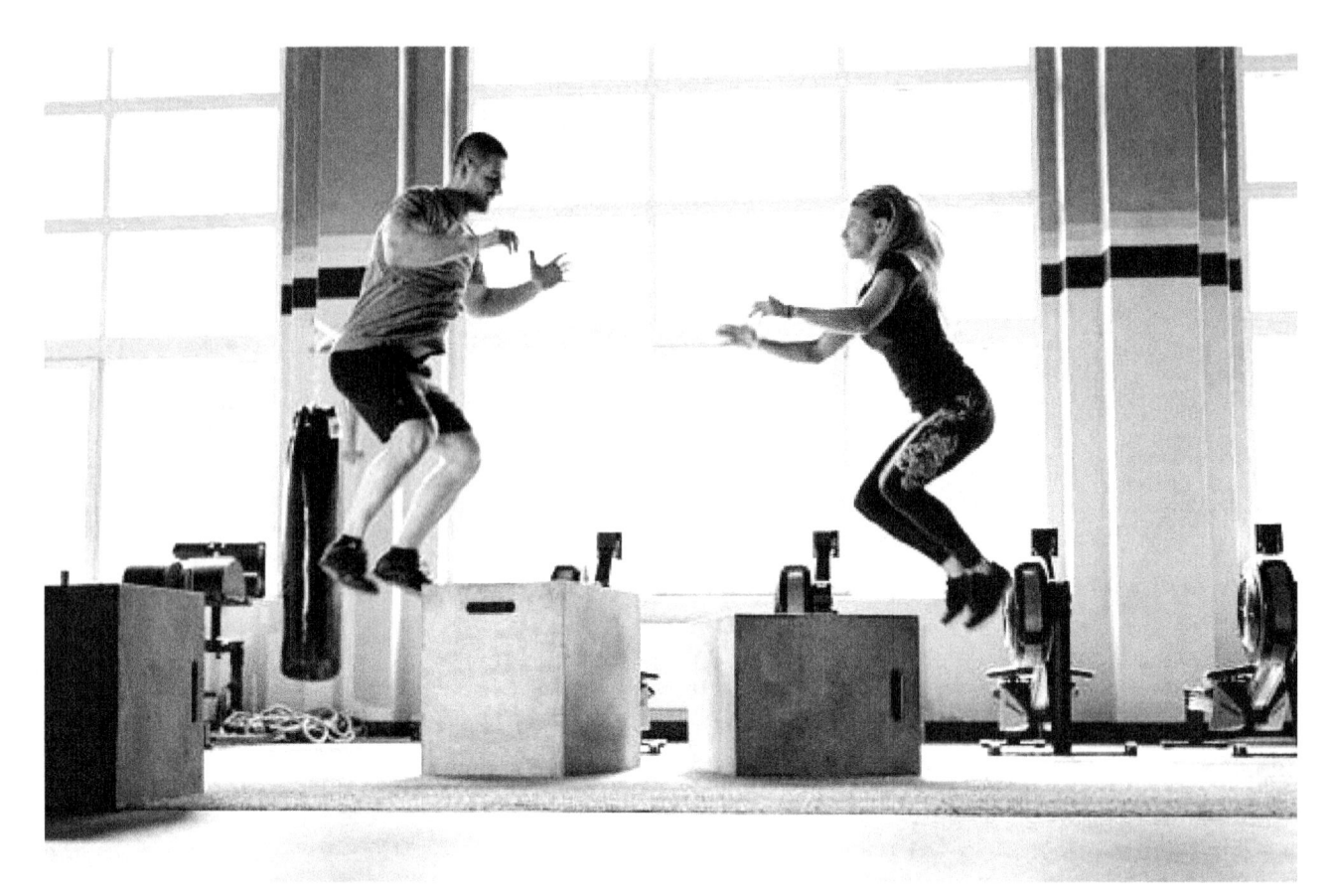

How effective are box jumps?

Box jumps are an incredible method for upgrading unstable power, further foster strength through your lower body, further develop vertical leap level, and for the most part work on athletic execution.

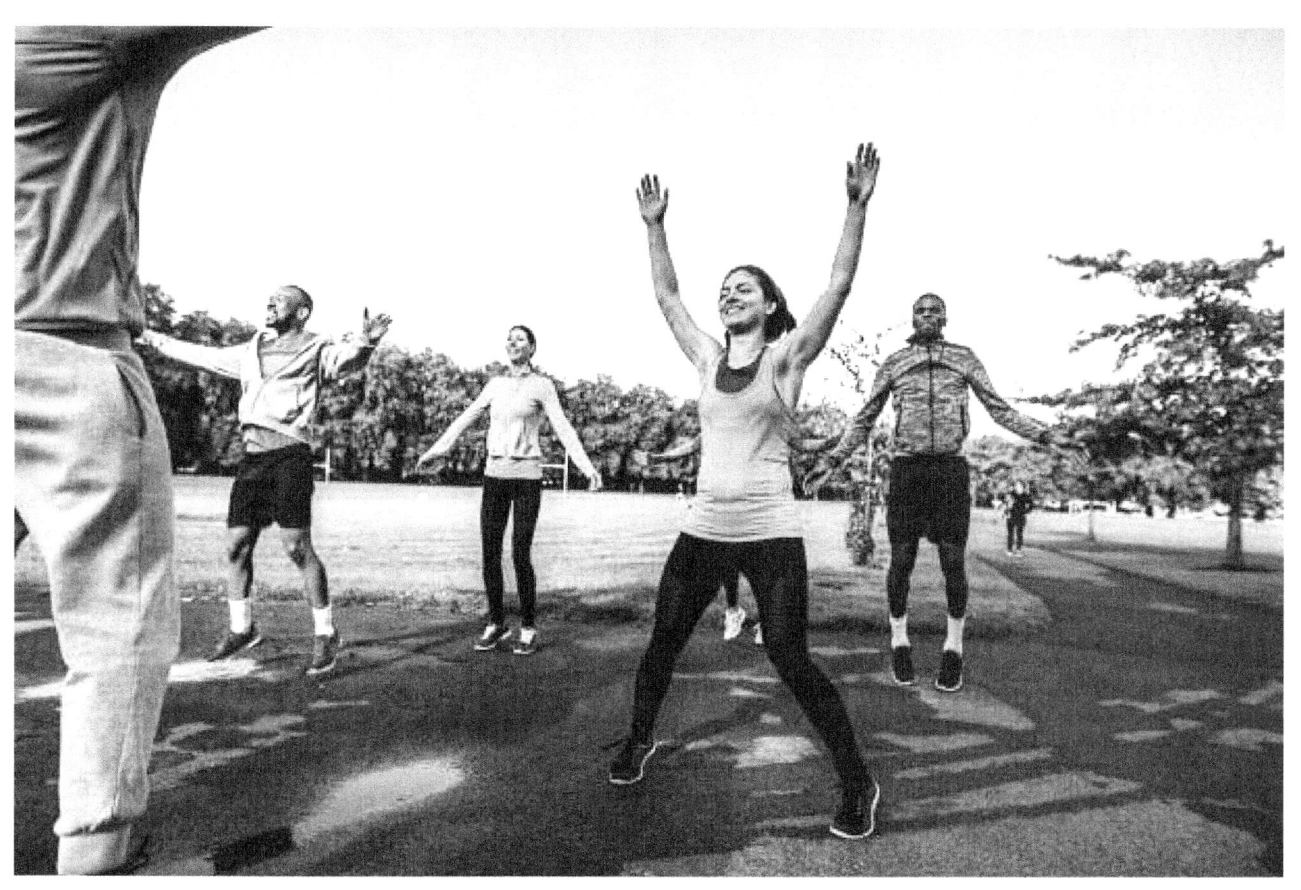

How effective are jumping jacks?

Jumping jacks are an effective all out body exercise that you can do anyplace. This exercise is important for what's called plyometrics, or hop preparing. Plyometrics is a mix of vigorous activity and obstruction work. This kind of activity works your heart, lungs, and muscles simultaneously.

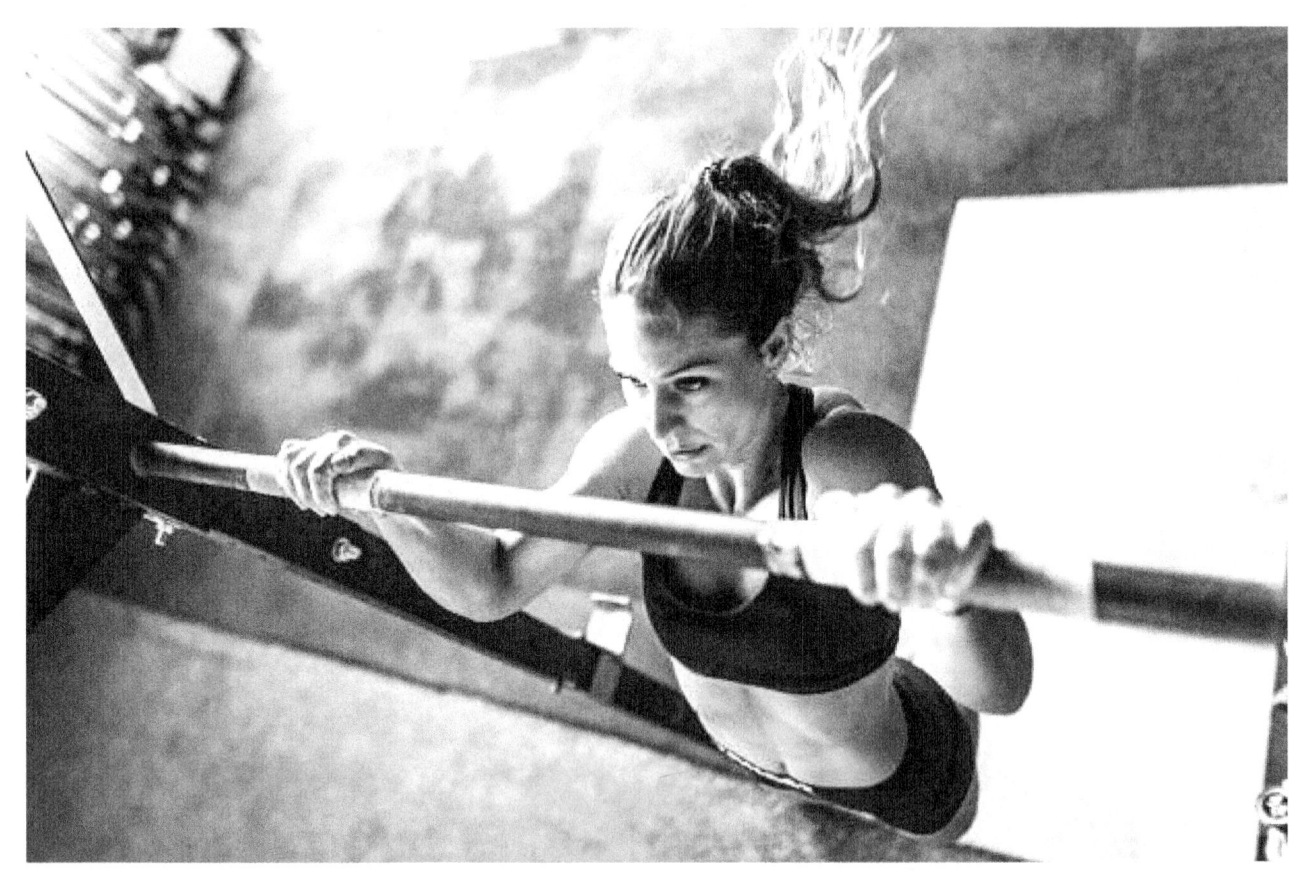

How effective are pull-ups?

The pull-up is one of the best activities for reinforcing the back muscles. Pull-ups work the accompanying muscles of the back: Latissimus dorsi: biggest upper back muscle that runs from the mid-back to under the armpit and shoulder bone. Trapezius: situated from your neck out to the two shoulders.

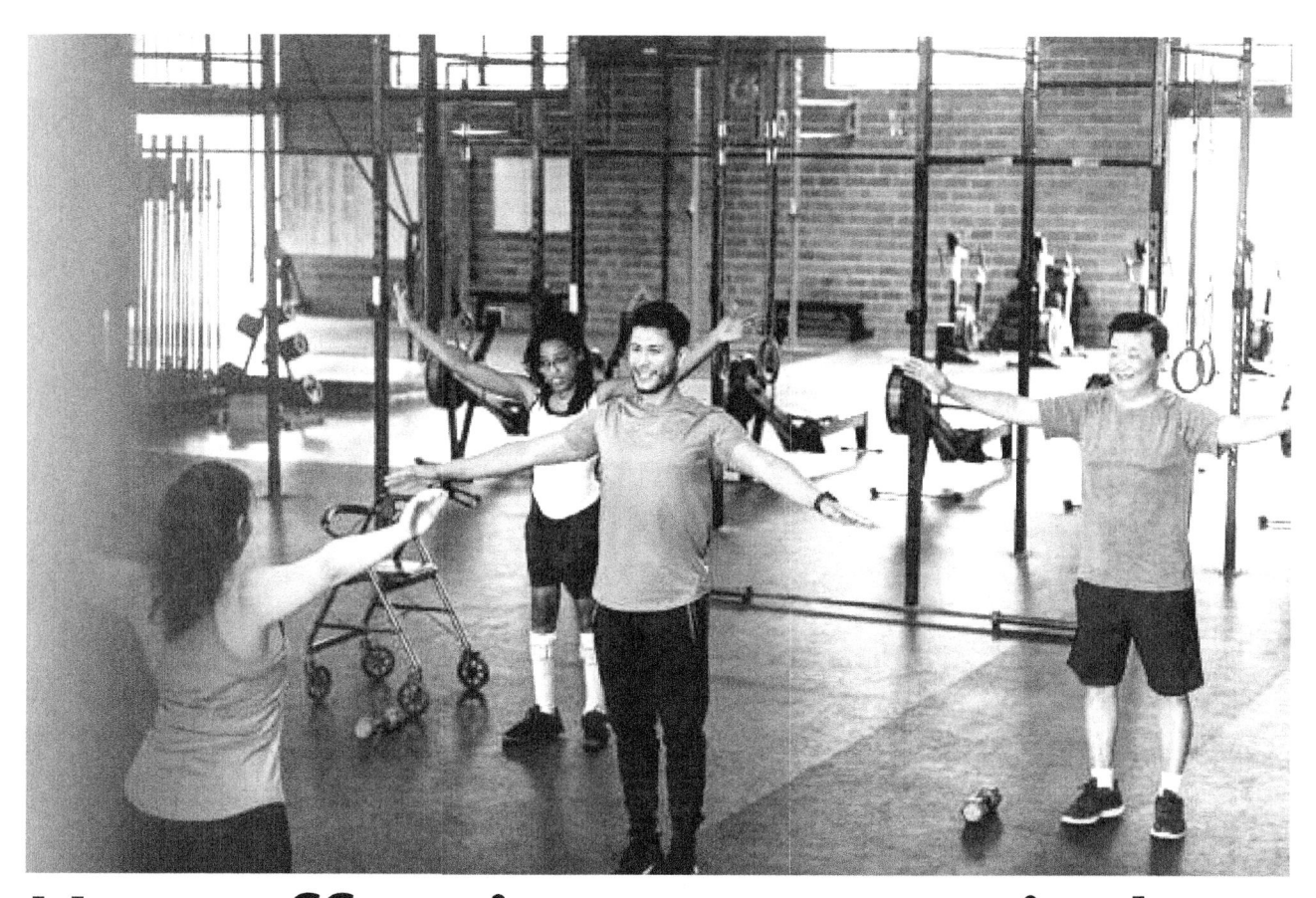

How effective are arm circles?

As well as utilizing your center, arm circles can truly deal with conditioning the muscles in your shoulder and arm like biceps and rear arm muscles. They likewise work on your upper back muscles, so they can be viewed as a full body exercise.

INCHWORM WALKING

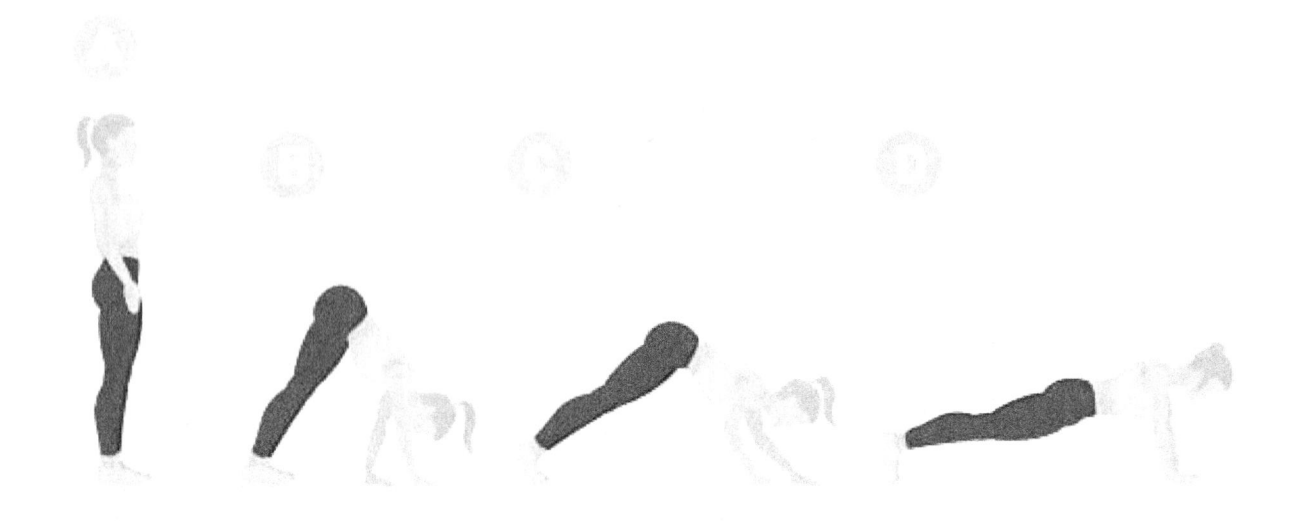

How effective are inchworms?

The inchworm is an incredible powerful activity used to heat up the whole strong framework. It centers basically around expanding adaptability all through ones hamstrings as well as increments strength inside ones shoulders chest and deltoids.

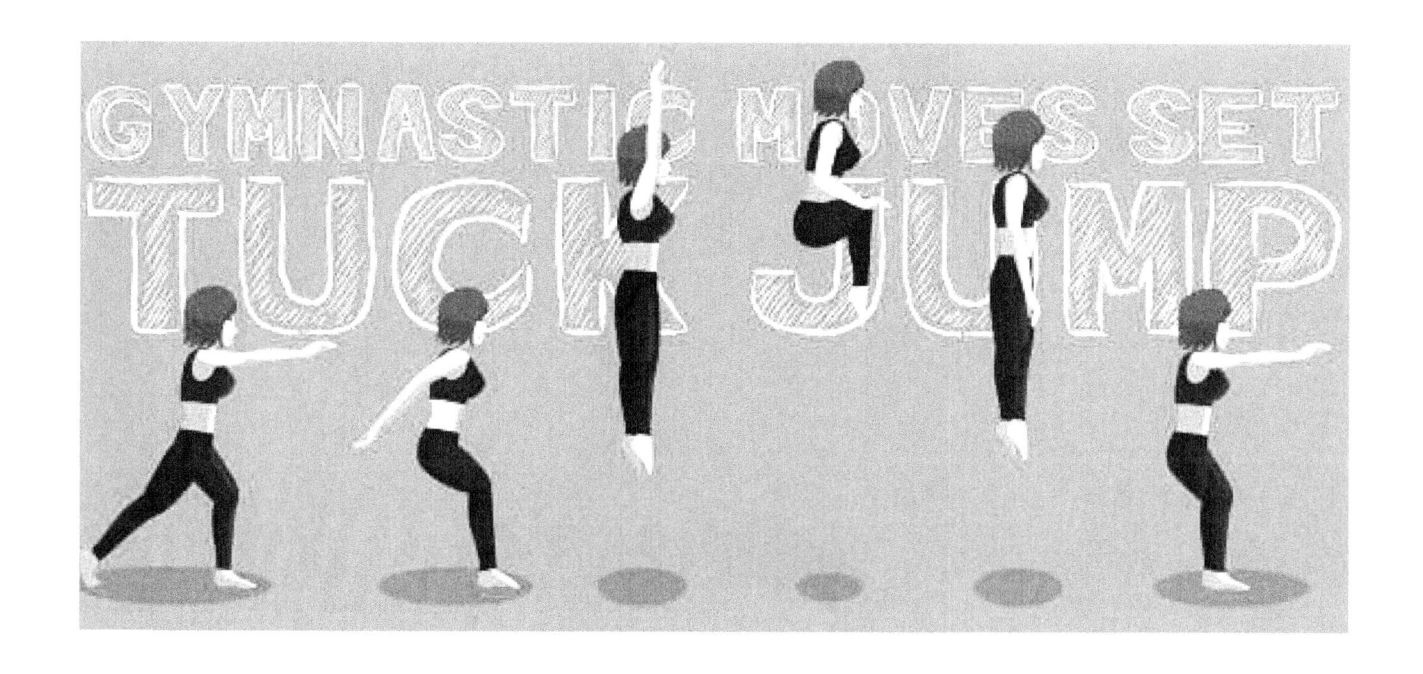

How effective are tuck jumps?

Tuck jumps are a sort of plyometric development, which can expand the pace of muscle withdrawal, increment power yield, upgrade muscle execution and at last outcome in improved athletic execution. They can be particularly powerful for sports like soccer and b-ball.

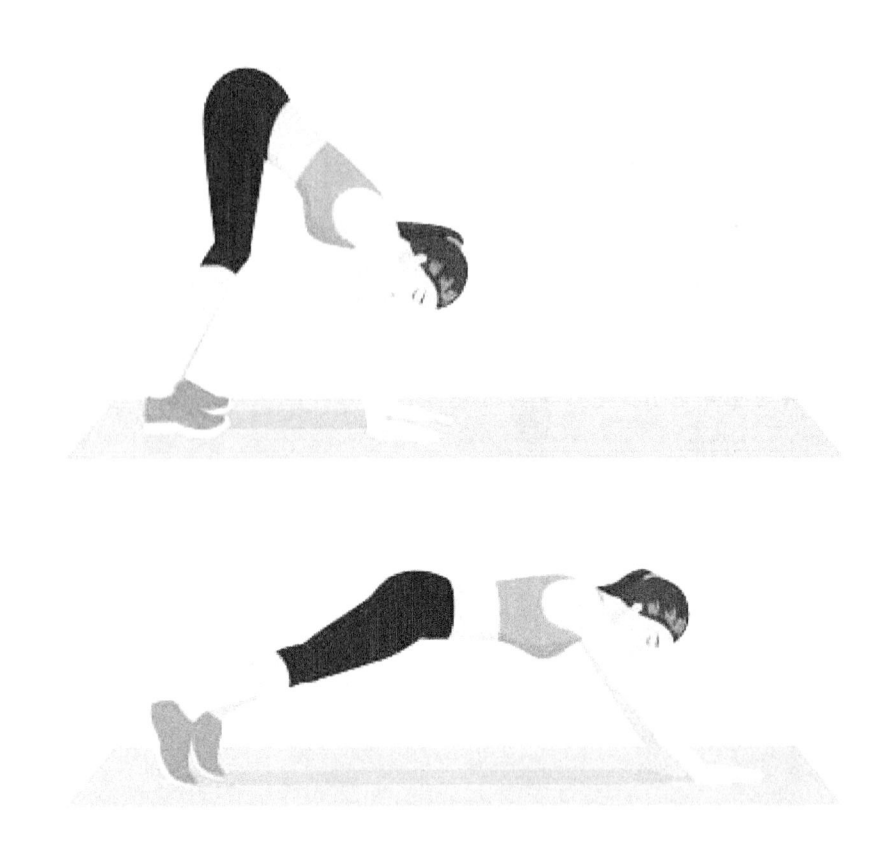

How effective are walkouts?

A Walkout is a plank variety that is progressively well known in practice classes of different types, because of its center and shoulder-fortifying capacity. While it's a full-body development, the leave chiefly focuses on the mid-region.

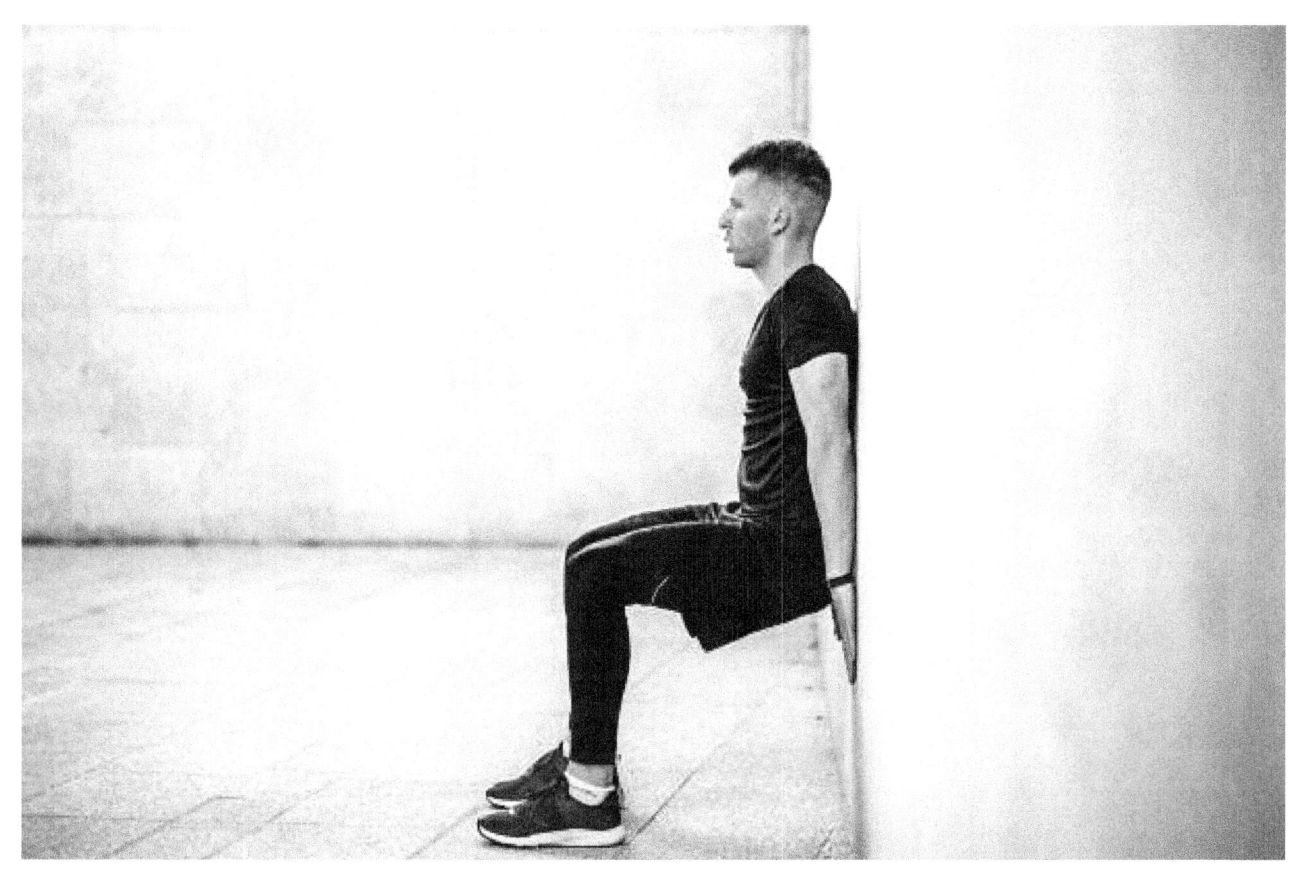

How effective are wall-sits?

Essentially, wall sit develops your isometric fortitude and perseverance in the glutes, calves, and quadriceps. Since a wall sit centers around the legs, it fosters its solidarity and steadiness. Also, as you probably are aware, our lower body is a significant region that aides in developing our general fortitude.

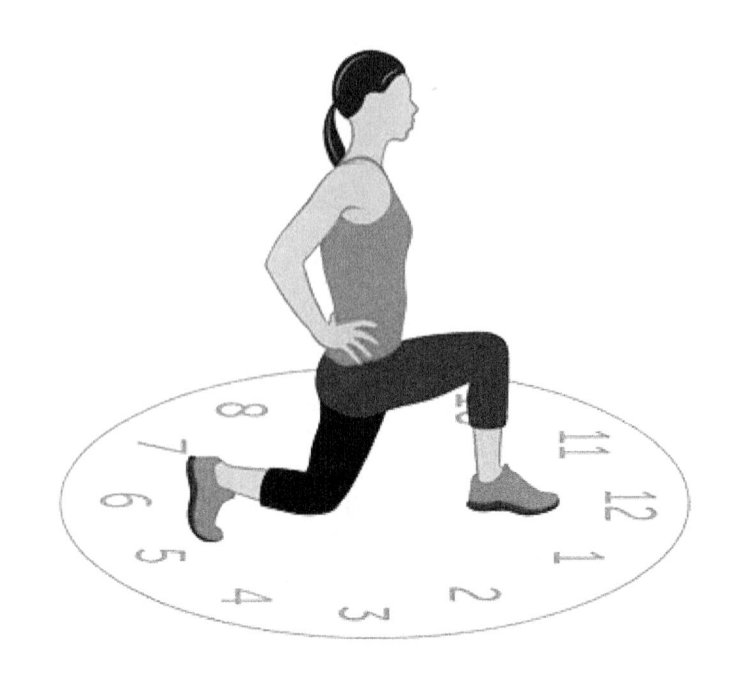

How effective are clock lunges?
The clock jumps fortify a wide exhibit of muscles in the accompanying regions:
Glutes.
Quadriceps.
Hamstrings.
Hips.
Thighs.

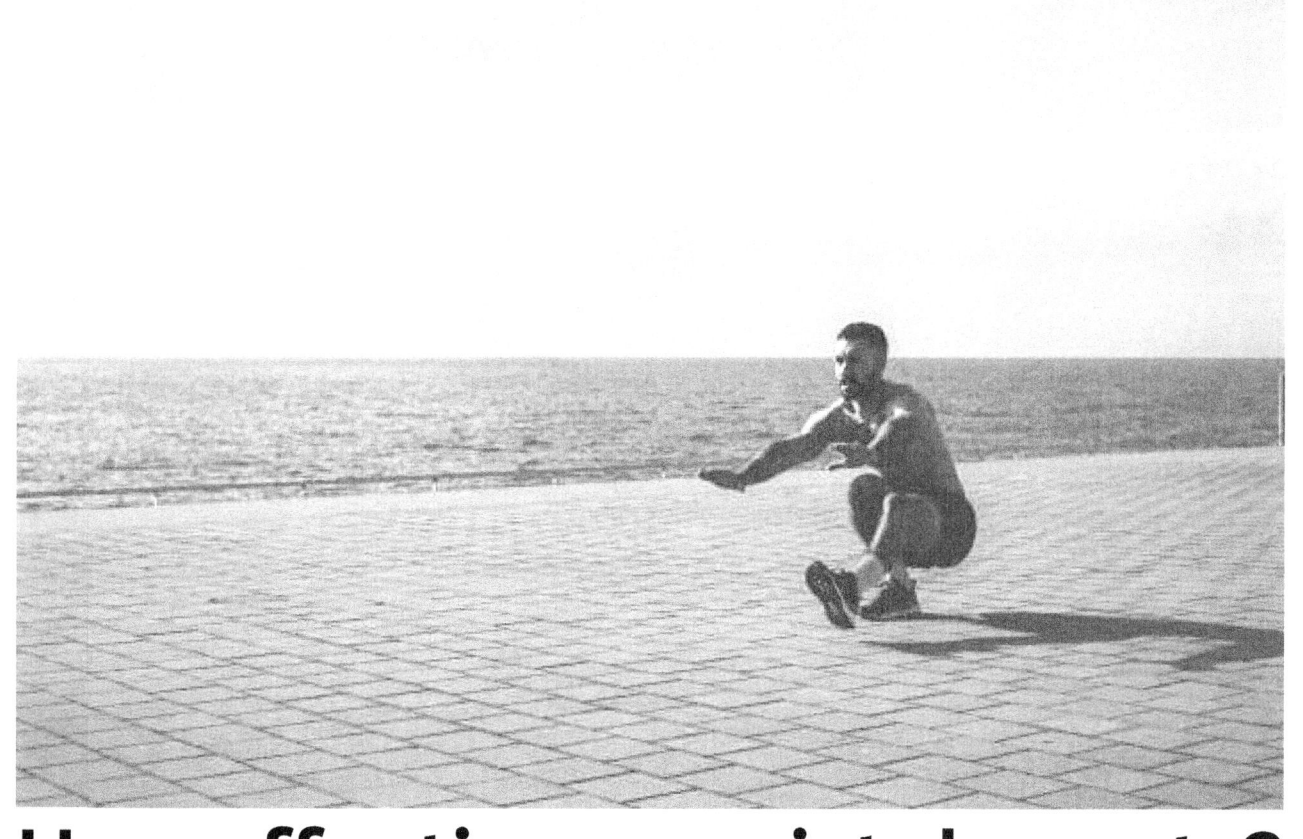

How effective are pistol squats?

Full scope of muscle enlistment. Further develops the back chain strength. Increment general adaptability and versatility along the back chain. Increments lower leg joint portability and adaptability.

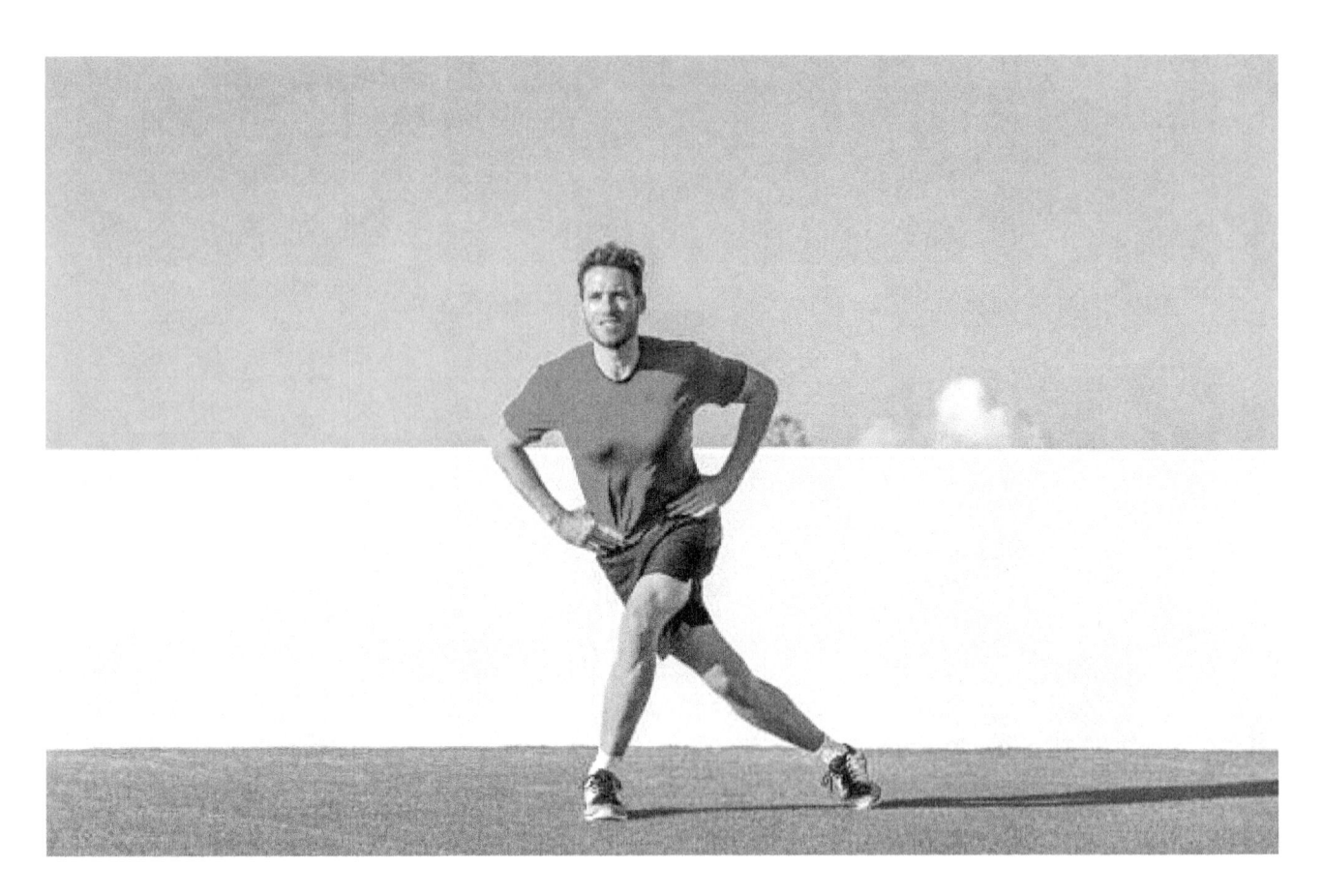

How effective are curtsy lunges?

Curtsy lunge is a viable and adaptable expansion to your lower body schedule. It focuses on a somewhat unique region of your rear than the customary rush. It centers around your inward thighs, gluteus medius, and gluteus minimus which works on your stance and balance out your hips.

Single-Legged Romanian Deadlift

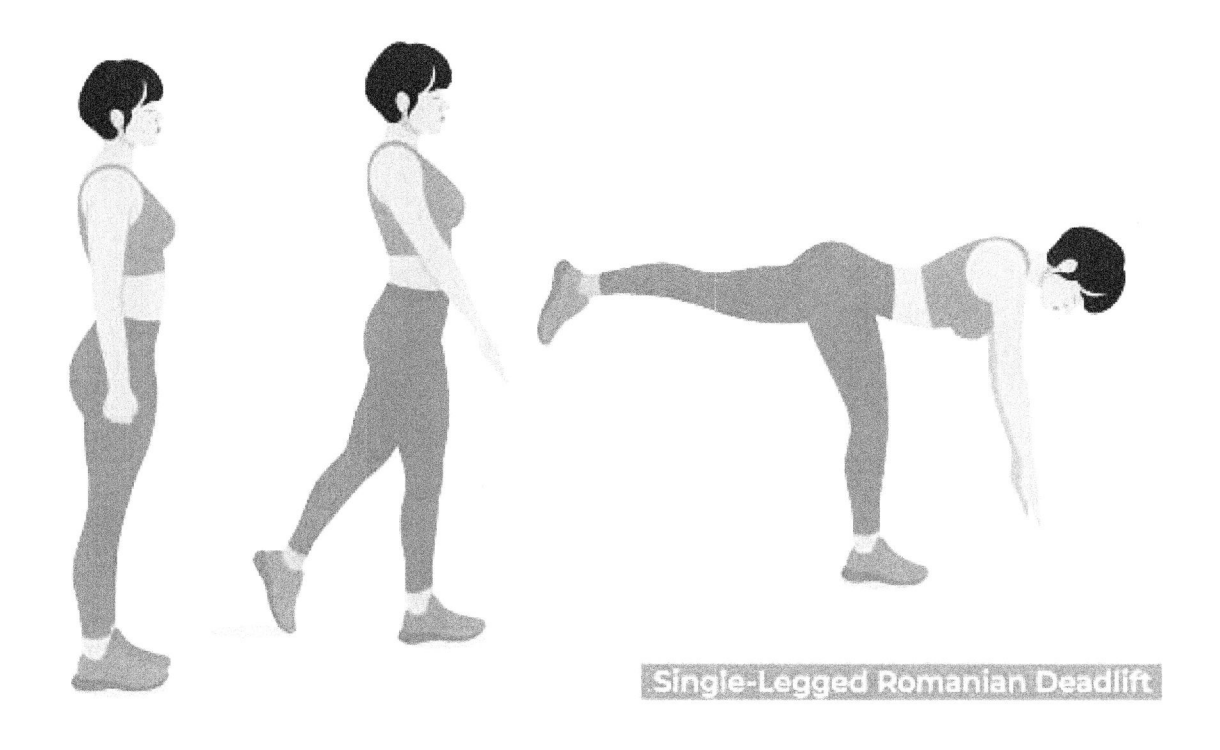

How effective are single-legged deadlift?

The single-leg deadlift is a basic yet successful activity for at the same time reinforcing and conditioning the butt muscles and further developing equilibrium. You can play out this with a portable weight or hand weight, in spite of the fact that fledglings can do it with no loads. You can make it a piece of your lower body stength and conditioning schedule.

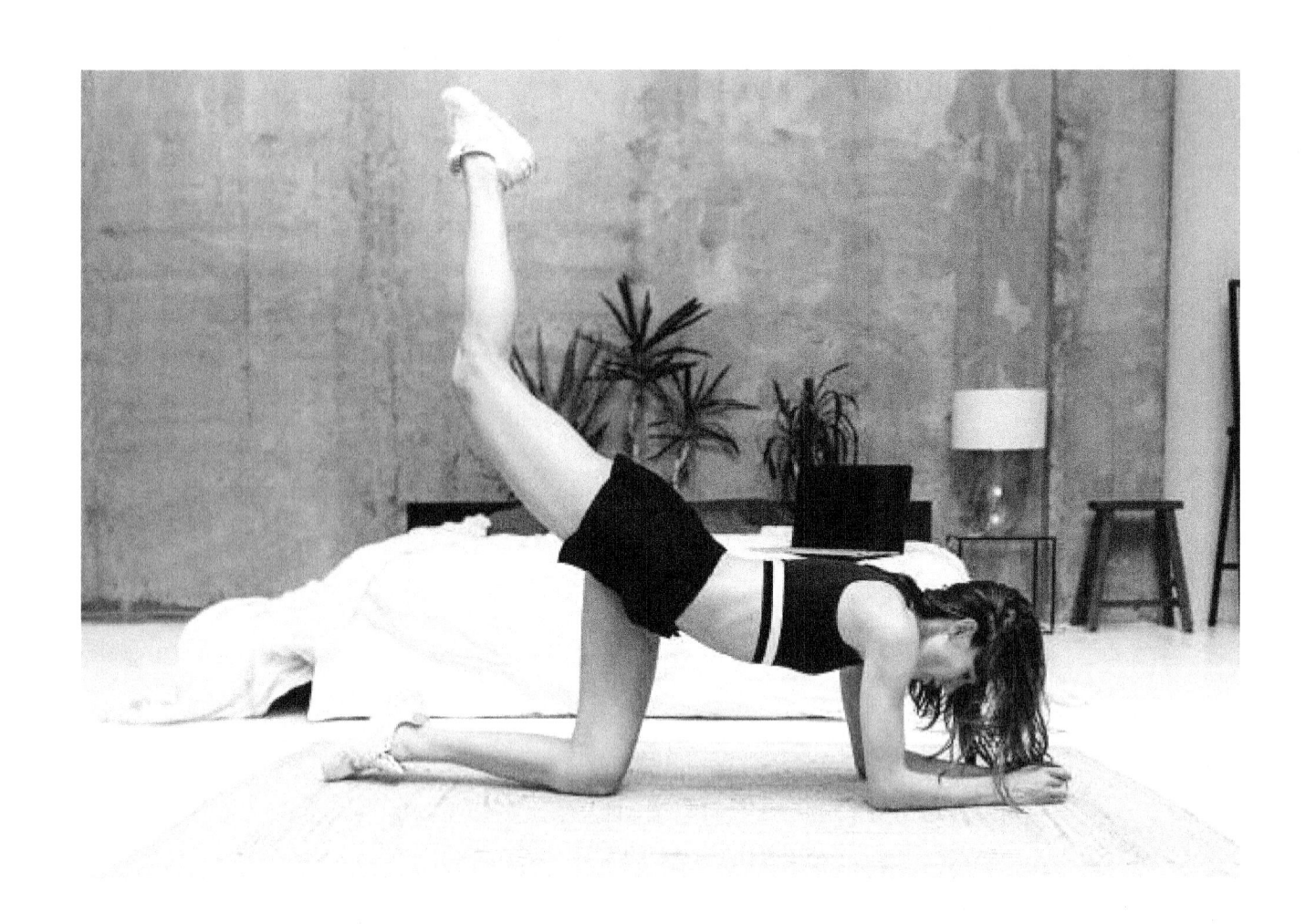

How effective are quadruped leg lift?

The quadruped is a bodyweight floor practice that reinforces the stomach muscles, lower back, glutes, and thighs and hamstrings. As it's a bodyweight work out, no gear is utilized as your own body and gravity give the obstruction.

DOLPHIN PUSHUP

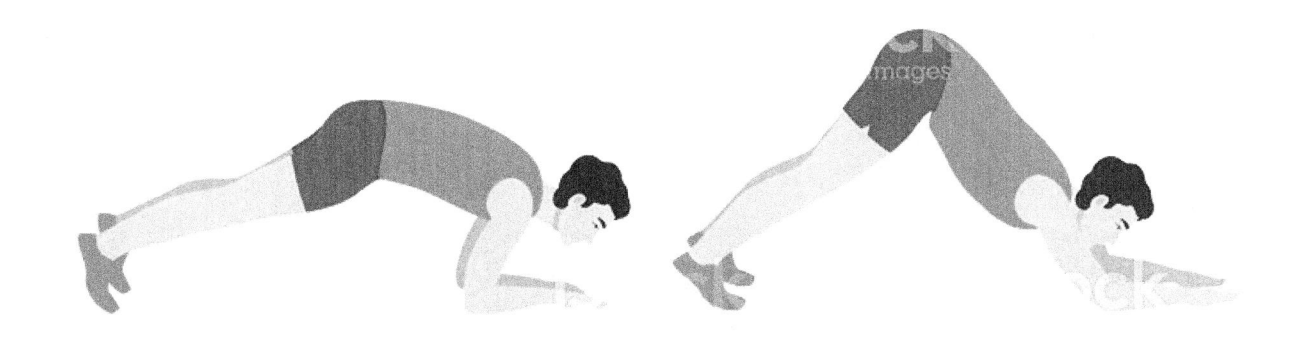

How effective are dolphin push-ups?

It is perfect for reinforcing your arms and shoulders yet you should utilize your abs and center muscles to settle your middle. The hamstrings and calves get a decent stretch. The chest area muscles that become possibly the most important factor in the push-up are the deltoids, pectorals, rear arm muscles, biceps, and erector spinae.

How effective are contralateral limb raise?

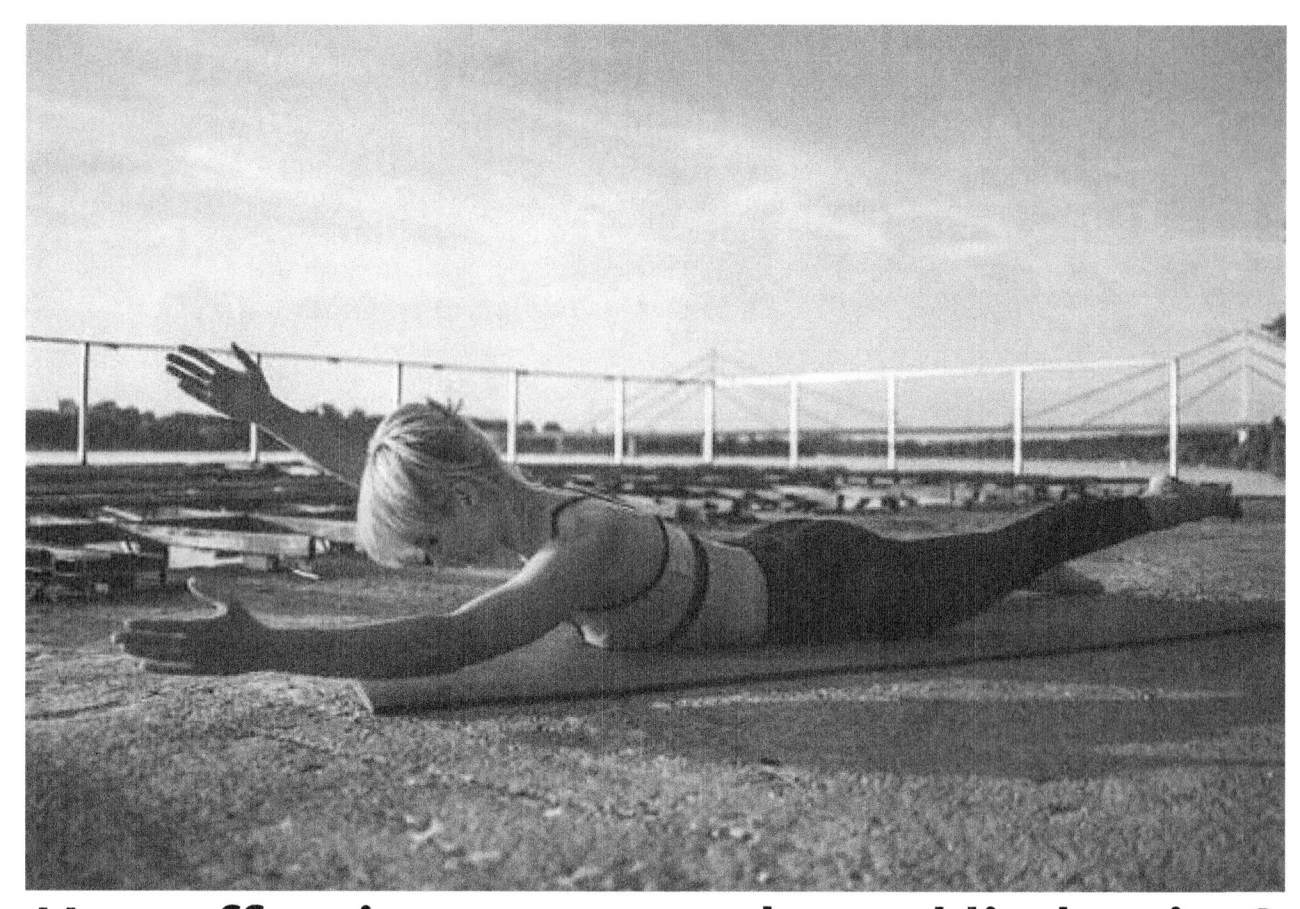

Contralateral appendage raises is an at-home work out practice that objectives glutes and hip flexors and upper back and lower traps and furthermore includes lower back and shoulders.

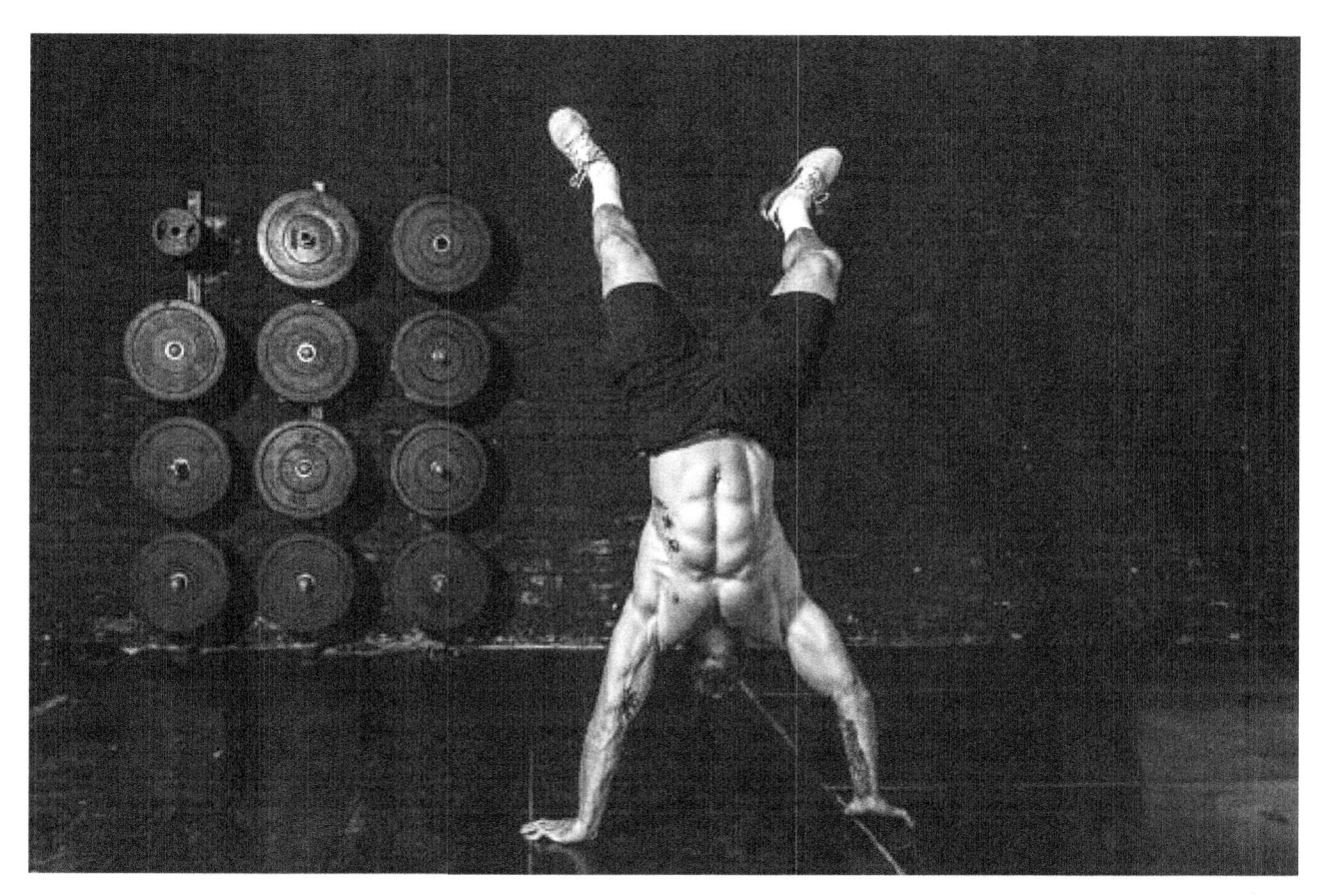

How effective are handstand push-up?

Handstand push-ups are a successful activity for building center, back, and shoulder strength.

There are a few advantages to performing handstand push-ups:

Handstand push-ups connect with different muscle gatherings.

Handstand push-ups don't need gear.

Handstand push-ups set you up for cutting edge strength-preparing works out.

Hindu / Judo Push-up / Dive Bombers

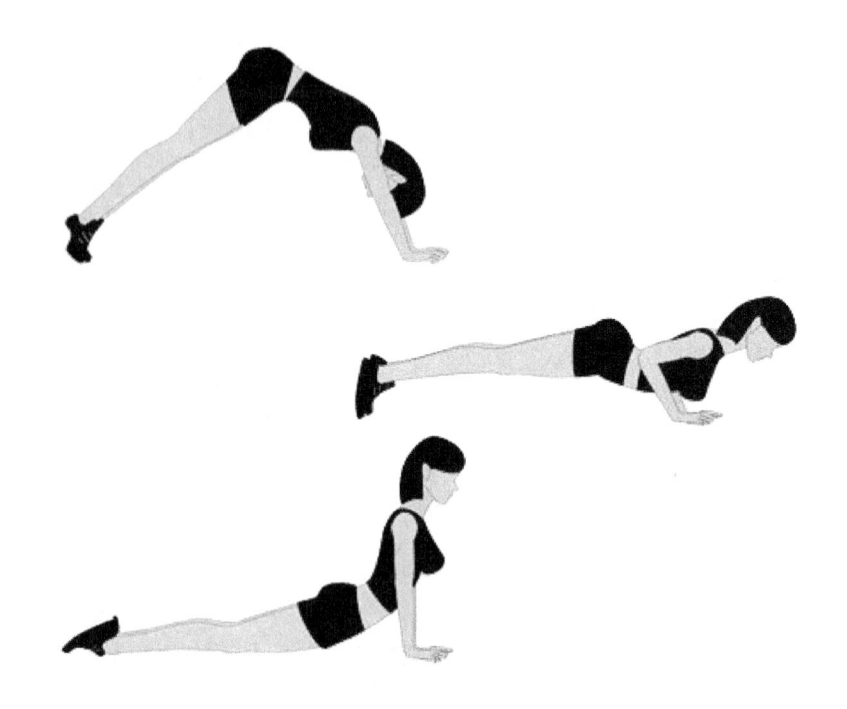

How effective are judo push-ups?

The judo push-up is a high level movement of the push-up that objectives the shoulders and rear arm muscles. The activity additionally further develops lower back adaptability

L-SIT POSITIONING CUES

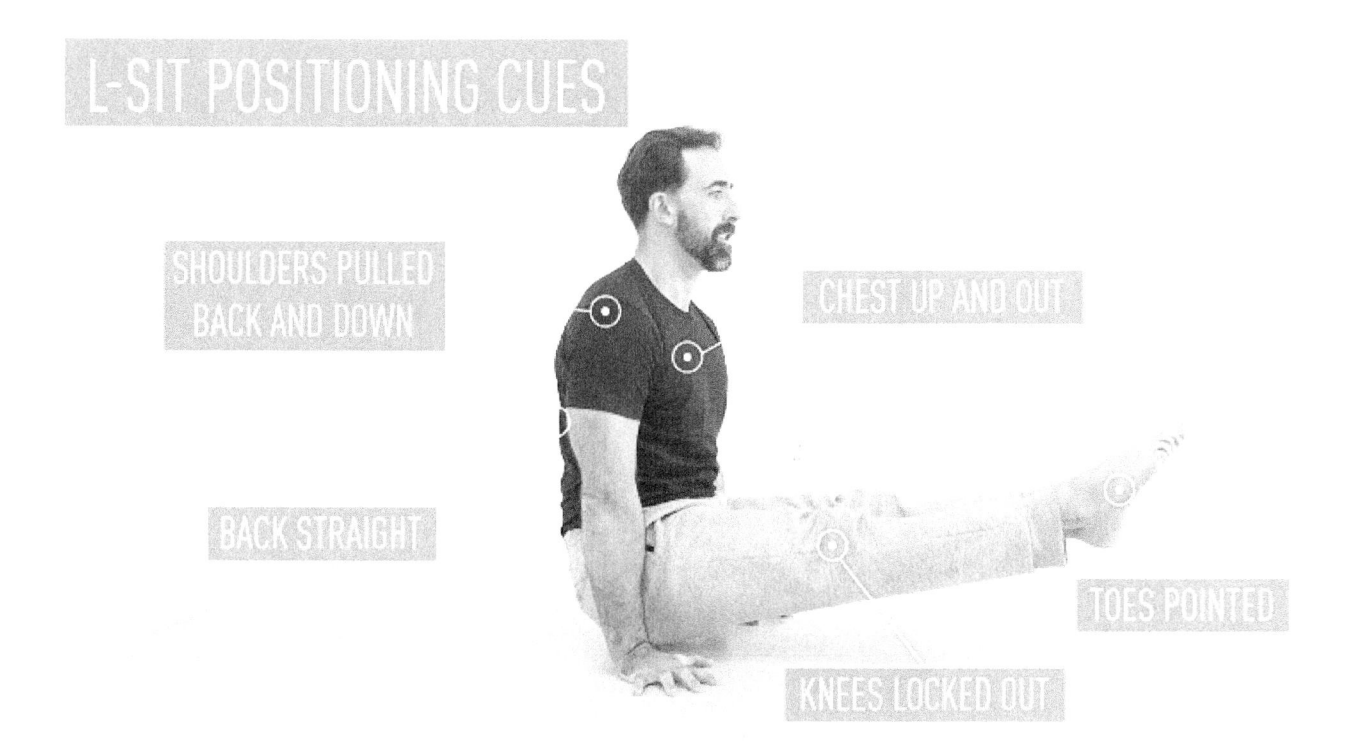

- SHOULDERS PULLED BACK AND DOWN
- CHEST UP AND OUT
- BACK STRAIGHT
- TOES POINTED
- KNEES LOCKED OUT

How effective are L seat?

Although the L-sit takes care of business with the stomach muscles, it is a full-body practice that draws in the quads, hip flexors, shoulders, rear arm muscles, and lats. The L-sit is a powerful activity for building abs and can be more secure than other center moves that include a lot winding or flexion.

FLUTTER KICKS

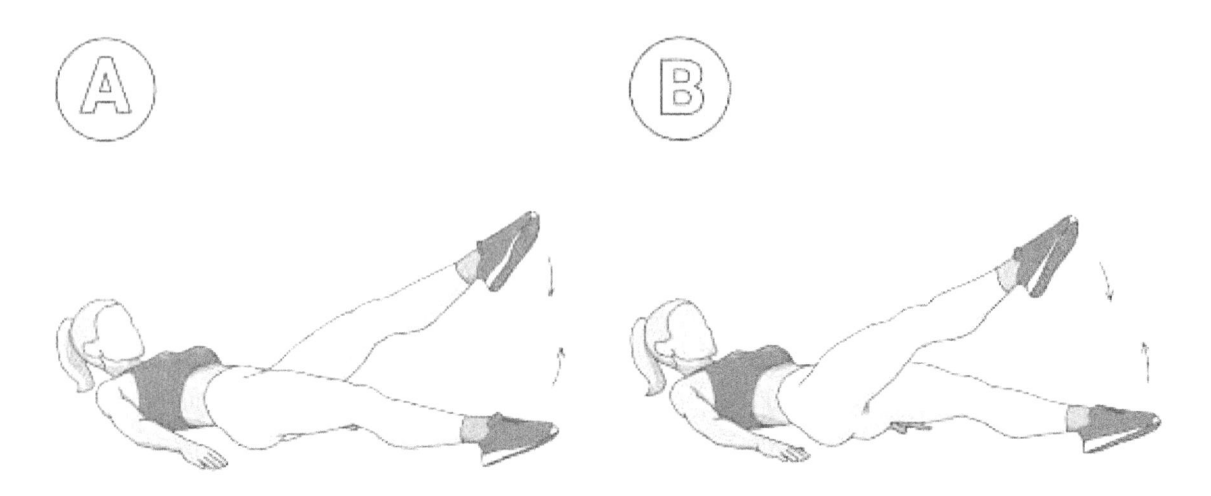

Ⓐ Ⓑ

How effective are flutter kicks?

Flutter kicks can be a low effect and successful method for reinforcing your center and work your lower abs, glutes, hip flexors, and quads. When done while lying on your stomach, ripple kicks can likewise reinforce your lower back muscles and assist with lightening back torment.

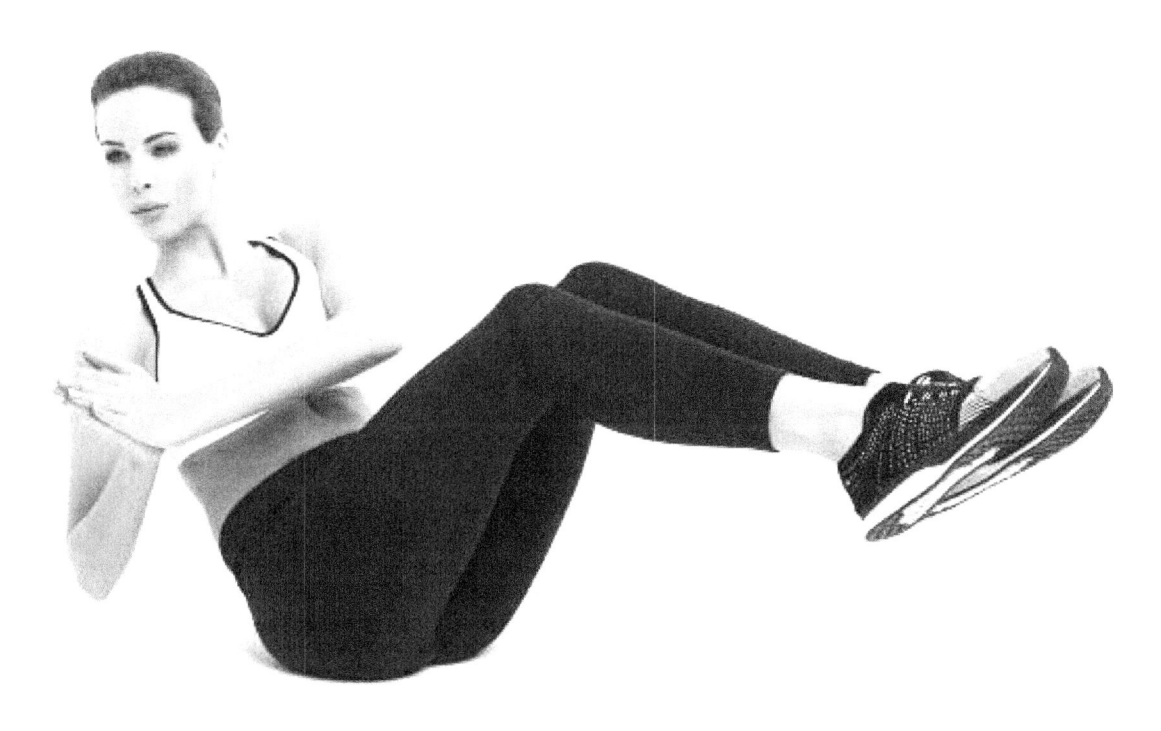

How effective are Russian twist?

The Russian curve is a viable method for building your center and shoulders. It's a well known practice among competitors since it assists with rotational development, which happens frequently in sports. It might seem to be a straightforward development, however it requires a ton of solidarity and backing.

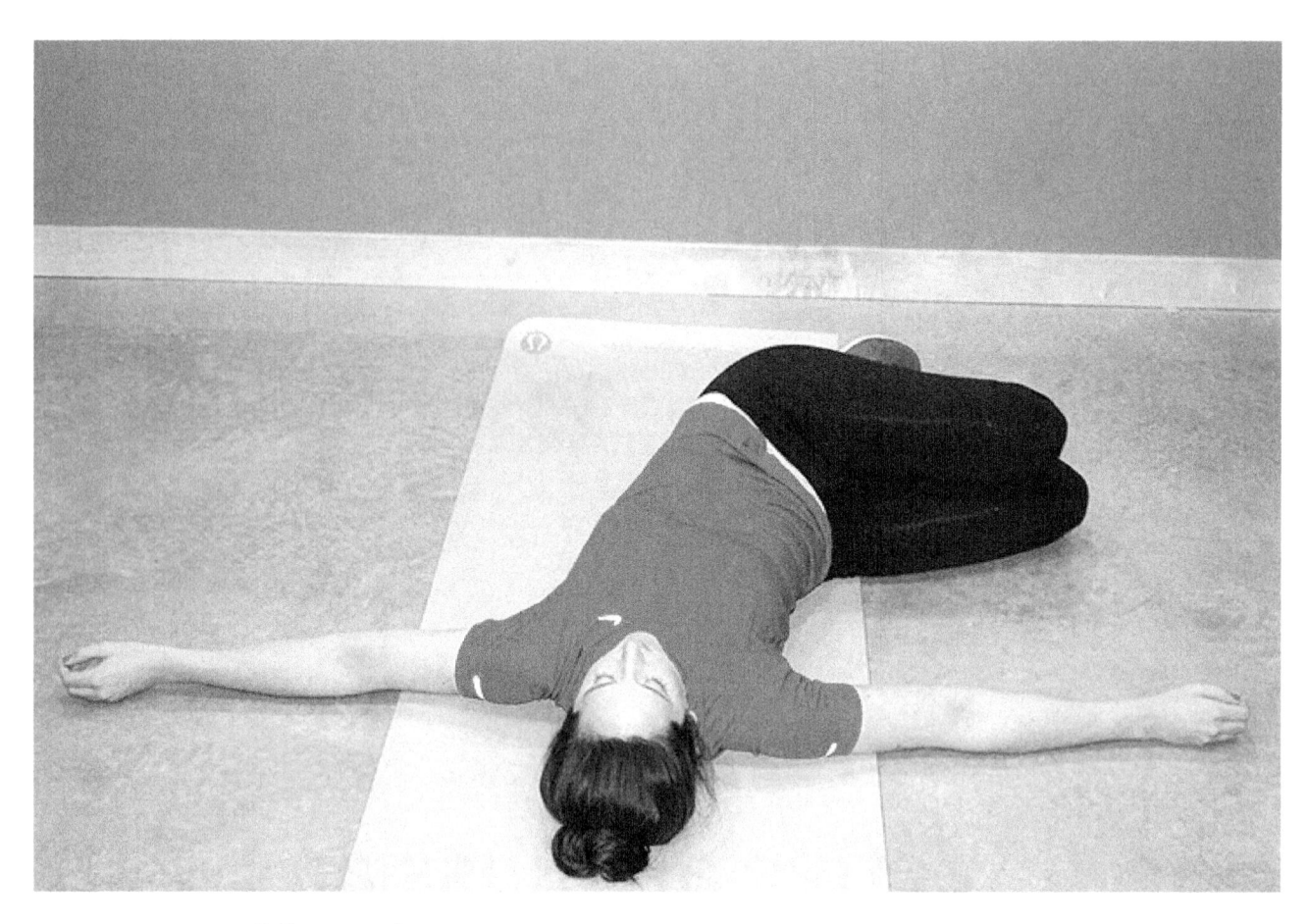

How effective are segmental rotations?

Segmental rotation is an activity used to further develop center strength, solidness, adaptability, and more noteworthy portability of the spine. The activity should be possible in different ways permitting you to advance, challenge yourself, and perform what turns out best for you.

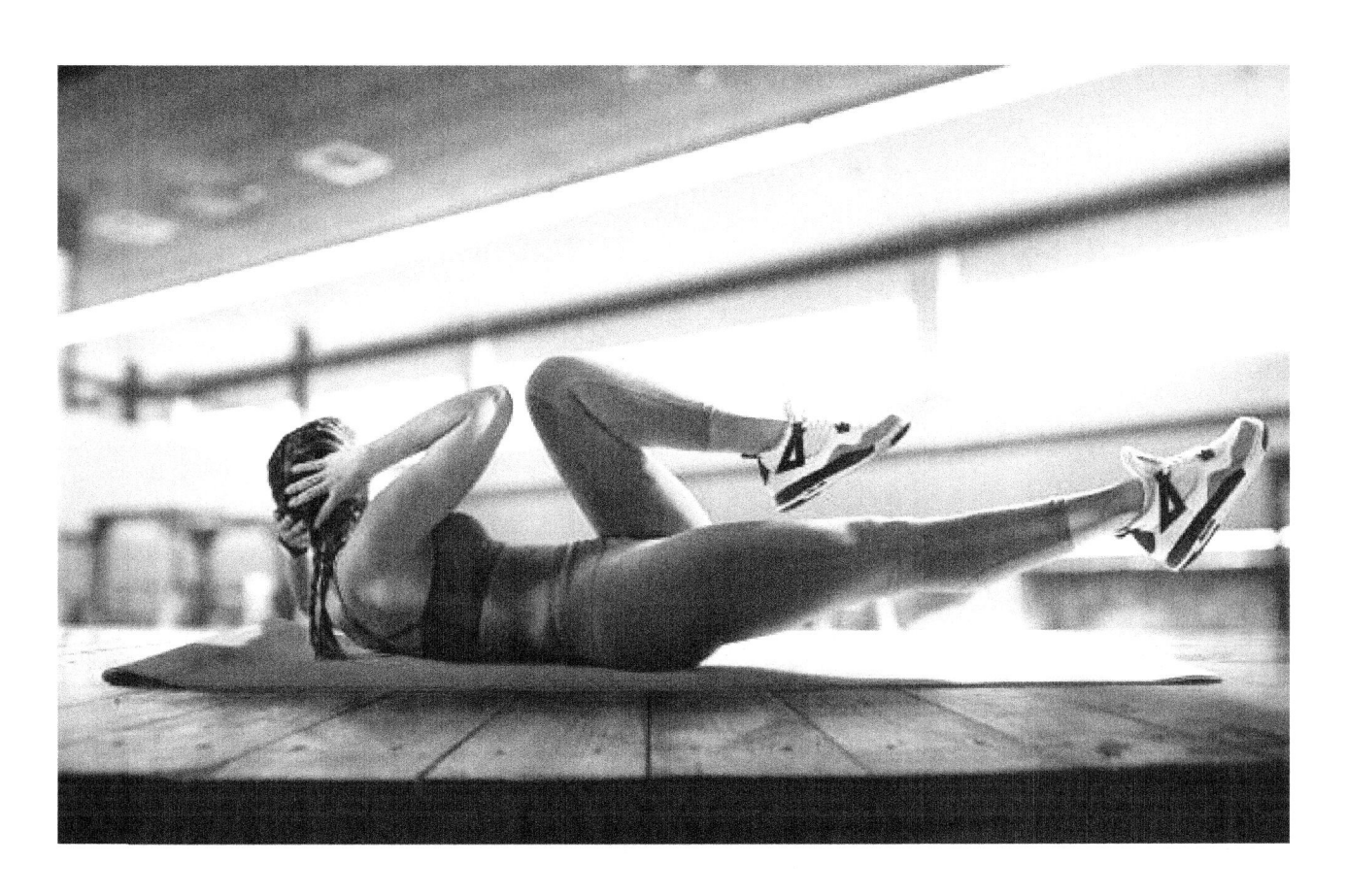

How effective are single-leg abdominal press?

Single-leg abdominal press stretch is a significant soundness exercise that stresses the abs. The abs work in different jobs to keep the storage compartment lifted, keep in touch between the lower back and the mat, and keep the stomach wall pulled in.

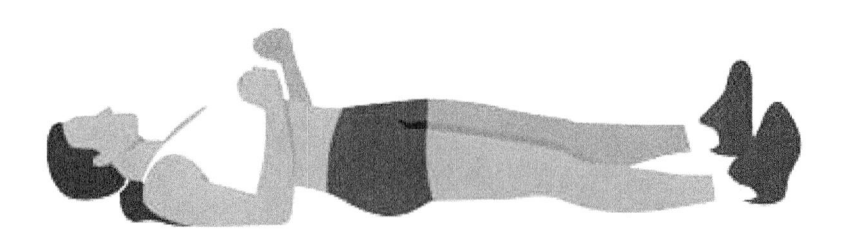

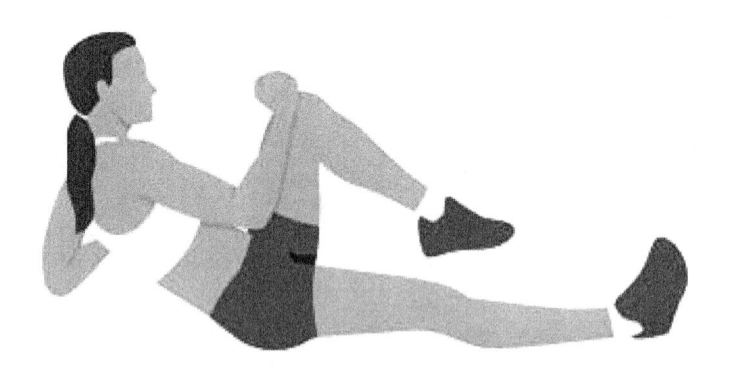

How effective are sprinter sit-ups?

Sprinter Sit-Up is an amazing center strength move that utilizations body weight alone to fortify and shape your paunch. Your fundamental old sit up is a dependable method for reinforcing your center yet the runner sit-up takes it up a score for an all the more remarkable, serious move!

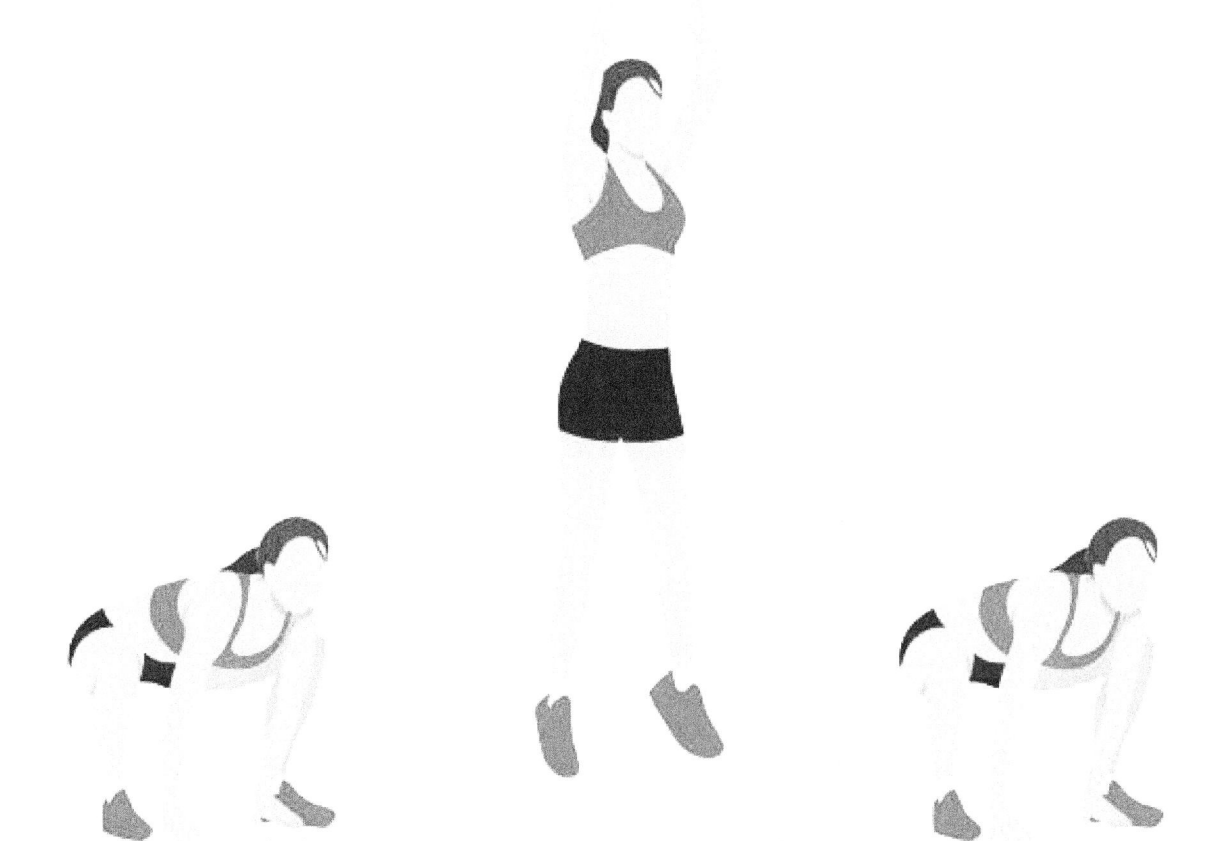

How effective are frog jumps?

With appropriate structure, frog bounces can build your pulse and work on your cardio wellness level. 2. Frog bounces fortify the muscles around your joints. The frog bounce can develop fortitude around your lower legs while likewise initiating your hip flexor muscles.

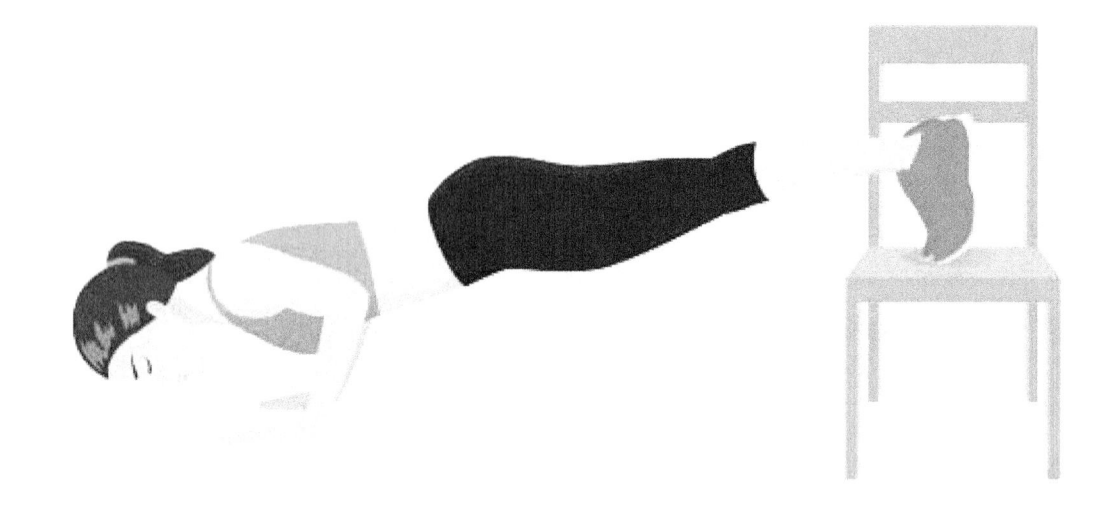

How effective are decline push-ups?

The fundamental advantage of doing decline pushups is areas of strength for building chest muscles. In a decay pushup, your arms push far up into the clouds from your middle. This development works your upper pecs and the muscles in your shoulders. When done routinely, decline pushups will assist with expanding your general chest area strength.

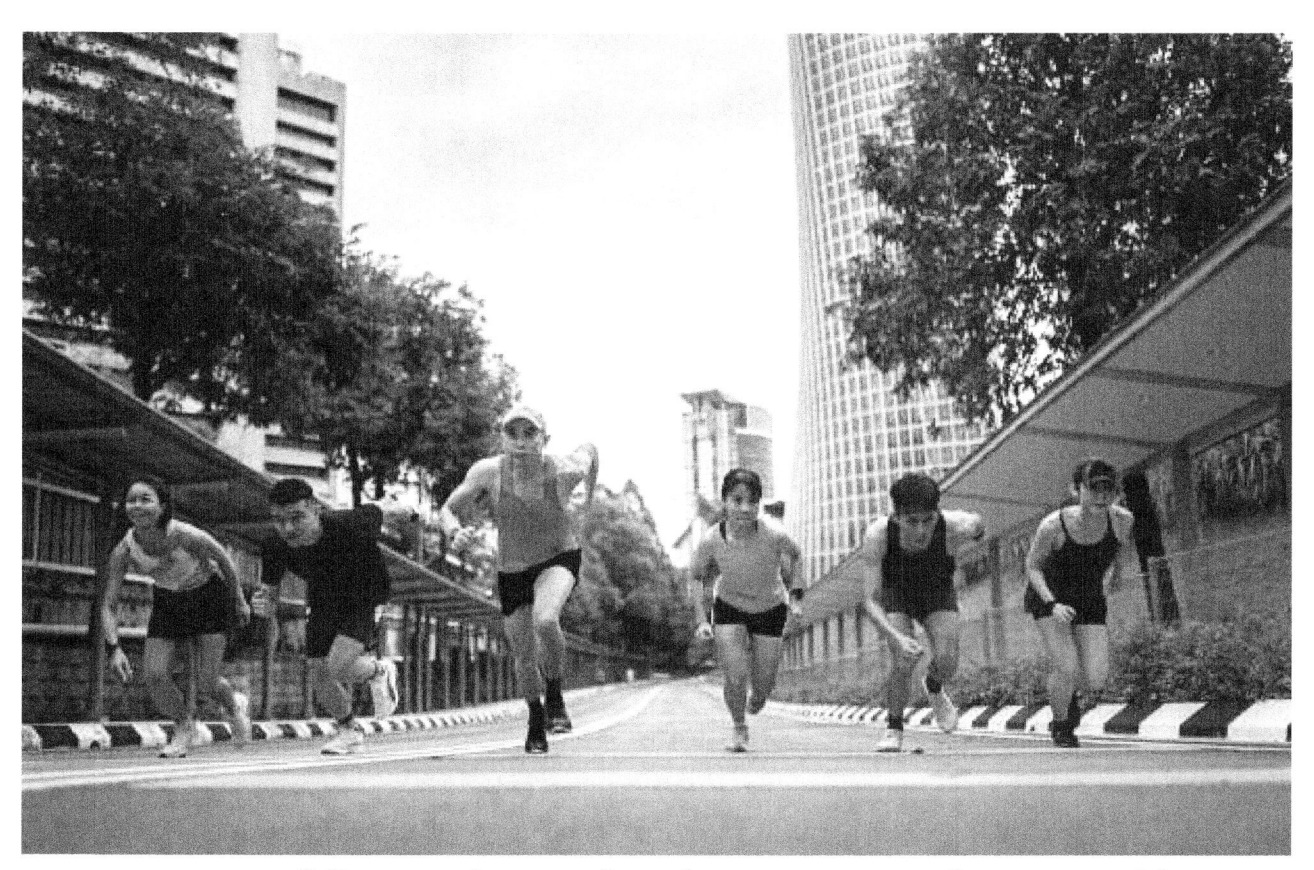

How effective is interval cardio?

Span preparing is the most effective type of cardio and can convey helps considerably more rapidly than regular cardio exercises. Research shows that 27 minutes of HIIT performed three times each week conveys similar oxygen consuming and anaerobic outcomes as an hour.

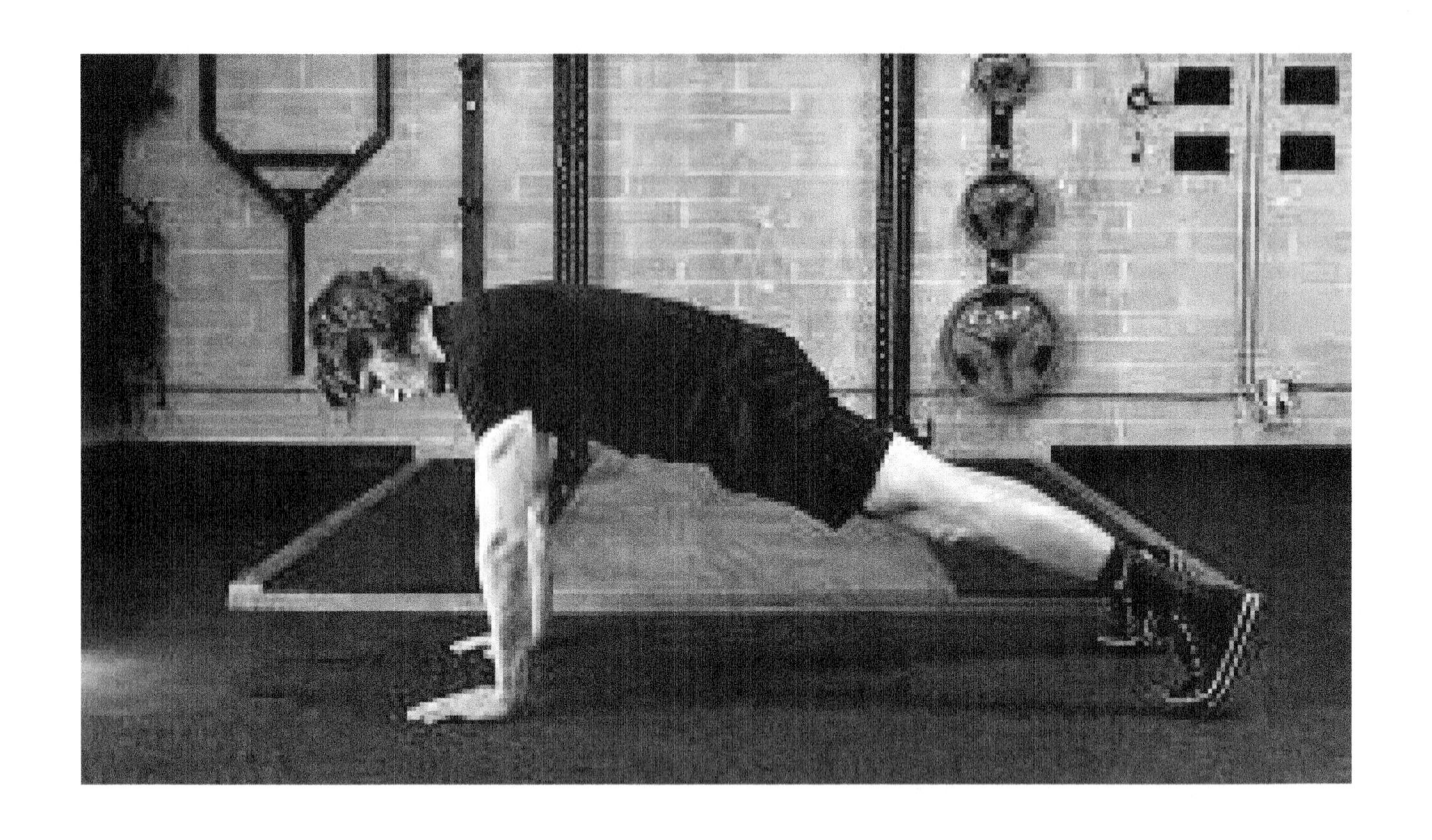

How effective are straight-arm plank?

The straight-arm board connects with the rear arm muscles and the center, being the most favored board drill for the individuals who will reinforce their chest area. In the interim, the lower arm board assists you with reinforcing the cross over abdominis muscle and turns out better for individuals who focus on their abs.

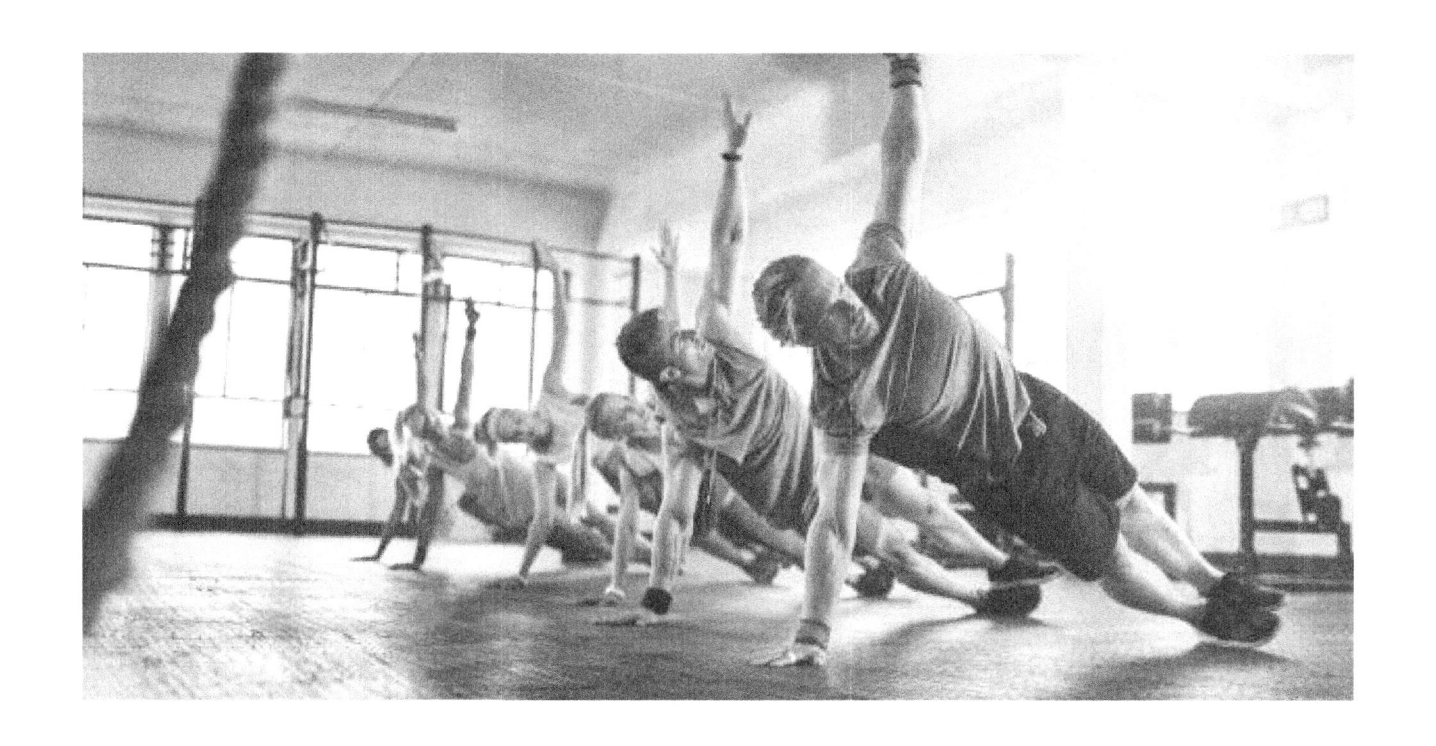

How effective are side-arm planks?

Side boards work the profound spinal settling muscle quadratus lumborum . Keeping this muscle solid can assist with decreasing your gamble of a back physical issue. Reinforces your center without focusing on your back. Not at all like crunches and situps, side boards don't come down on your lower back.

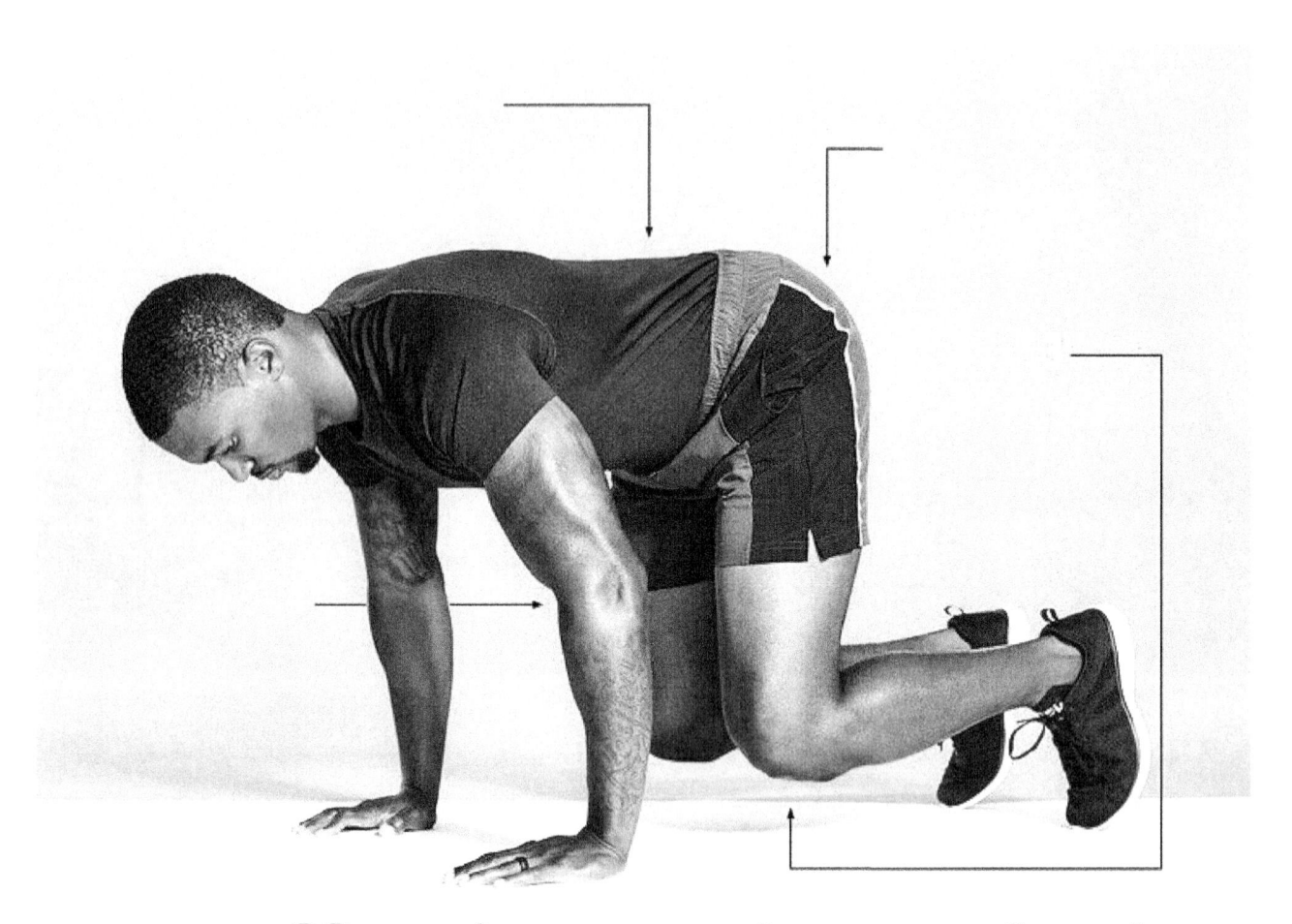

How effective are bear planks?

In general, bear boards are more compelling at further developing steadiness and execution, as well as diminishing injury risk and persistent low back torment, than numerous other stomach muscle works out. Consider adding one of the bear board varieties to your center preparation schedule.

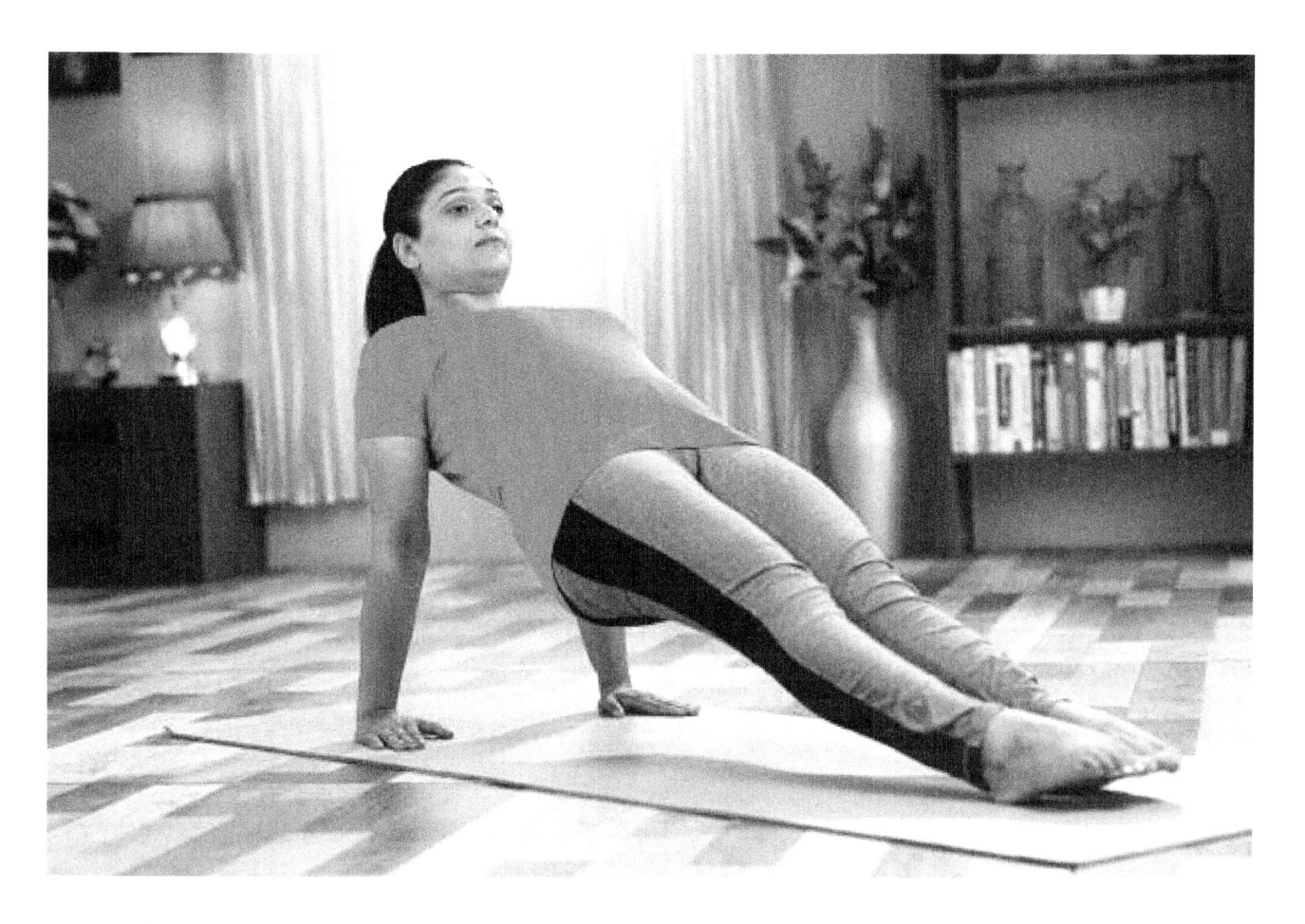

How effective are reverse planks?

Like all plank varieties, the reverse plank is an astounding method for reinforcing your center. It's particularly great for the muscles in your lower back, your hamstrings and your glutes, however in the event that you are appropriately propped, your abs will likewise feel the squeeze.

PLANK JACKS
WITH RESISTANCE BAND

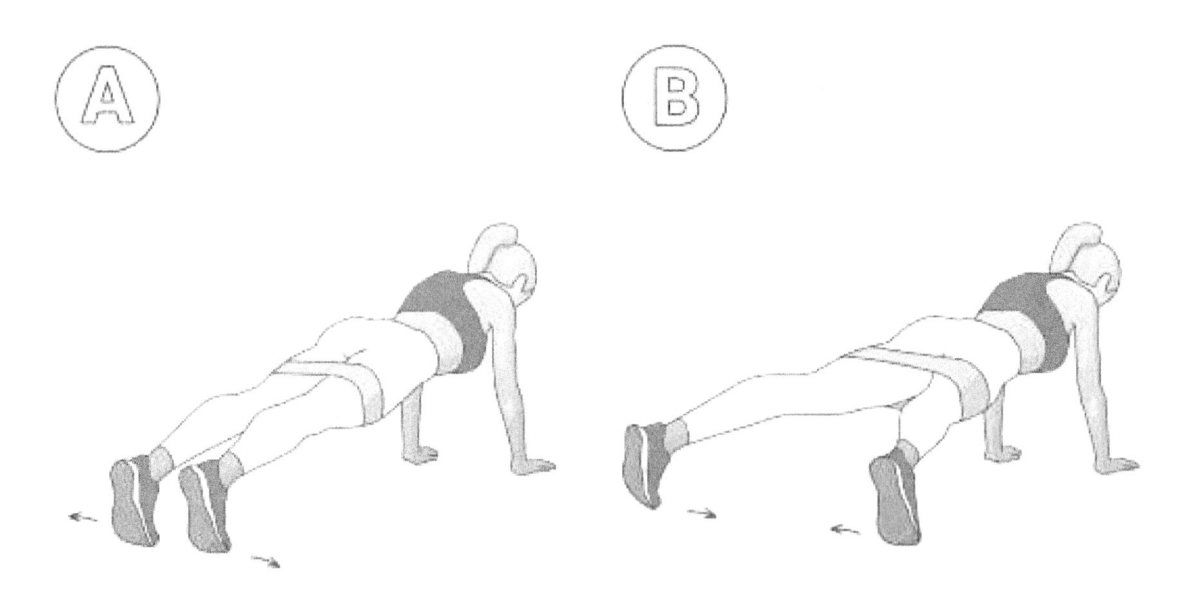

(A) (B)

How effective are plank jacks?

Plank jacks are a combined cardio and core-strengthening exercise. They can help you strengthen the muscles of both the upper and lower body. Adding plank jacks to your exercise routine a few times a week may also increase core strength and stability, burn calories, and help reduce fat.

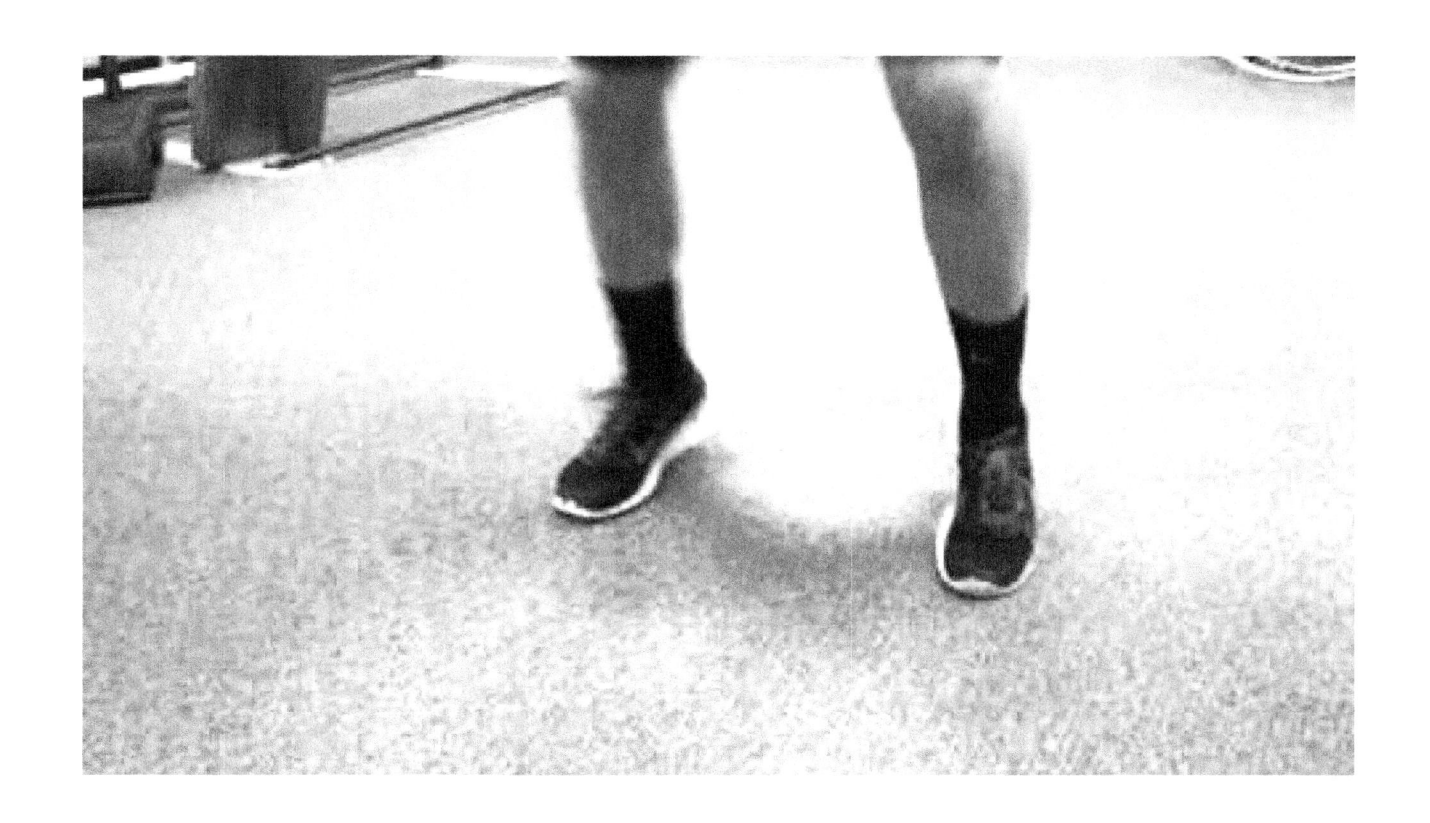

How effective are quick toes?

The fast feet is an incredible activity in the event that you want to work on your speed and deftness. This exercise builds your pulse and gives you an extraordinary cardio exercise. In the event that you're attempting to consume a few calories while working your lower body, you ought to add this activity to your gym routine everyday practice.

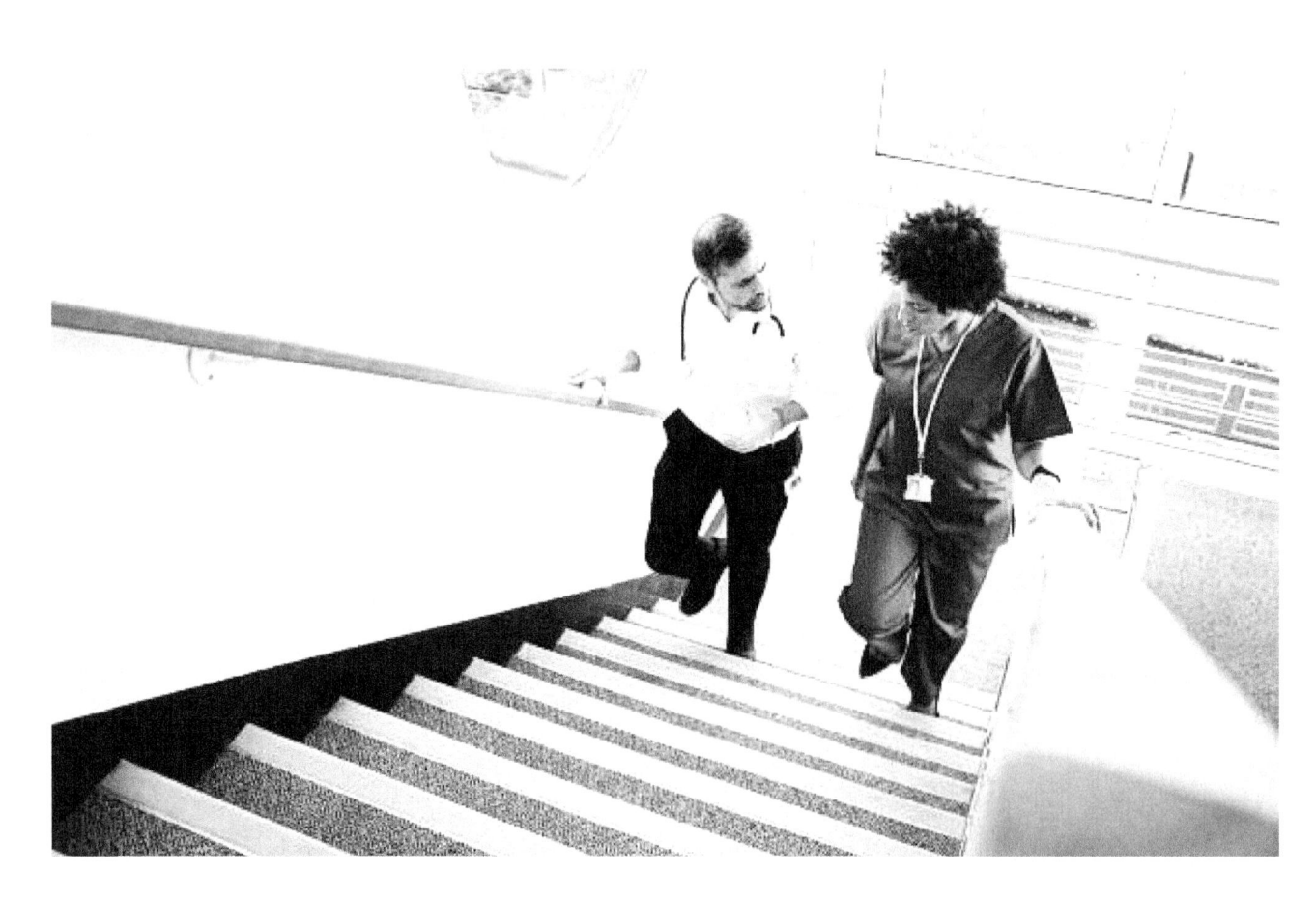

How effective is climbing stairs?

Climbing steps is one of the most amazing activities with regards to unadulterated FAT Consume, fortifying the lower body, conditioning the butt, thighs, calves, losing creeps from those cushy layers and gut and building incredible abs. Alongside these advantages is the massive great it accomplishes for your lungs and cardio vascular framework.

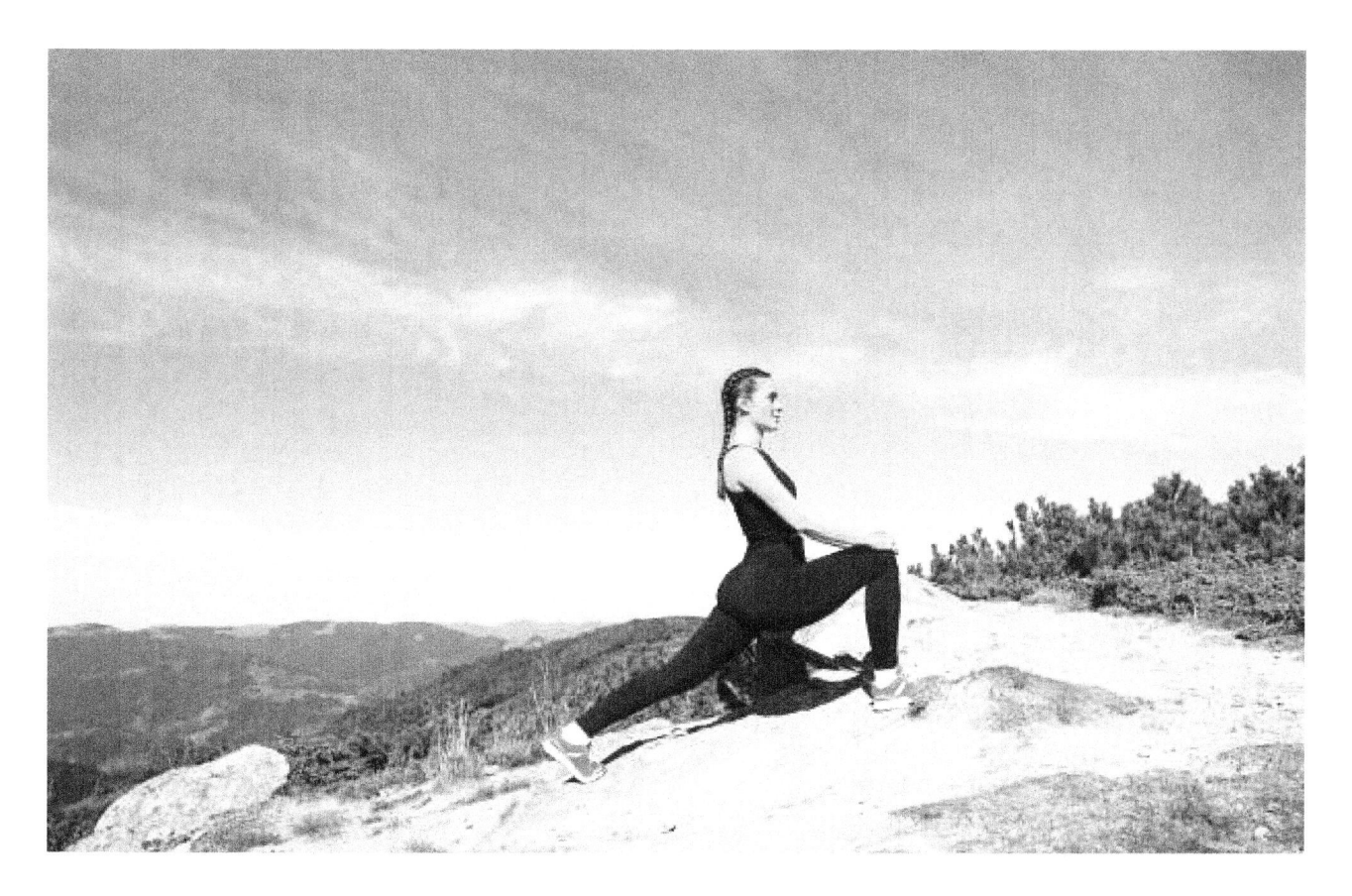

How effective are hill lunges?

The motivation behind why hill lunges are so powerful is that you are utilizing the huge muscle gatherings of your legs, glutes and center against the powers of gravity, which not just shapes your muscles, it builds your pulse for a fantastic cardio impact — which will consume calories and burn fat!

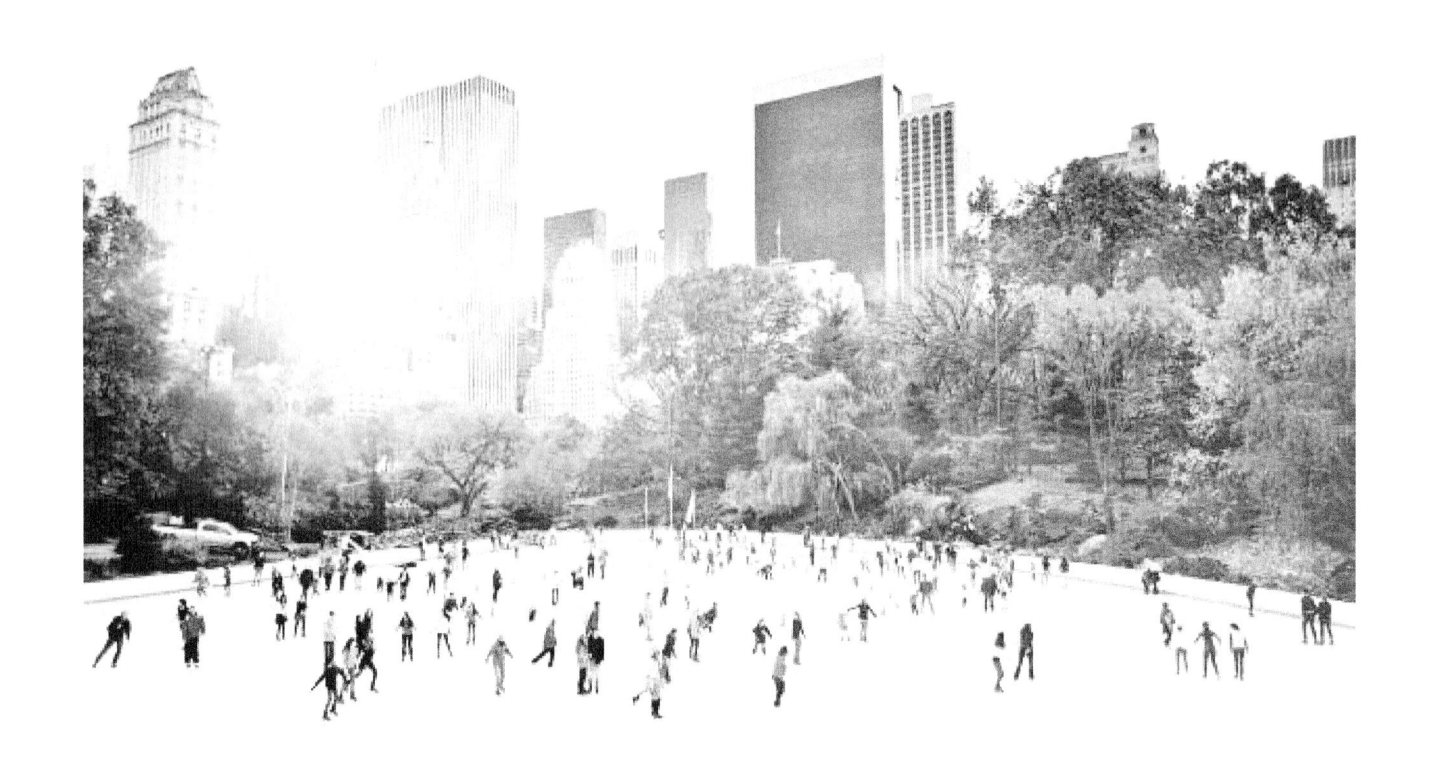

How effective is ice skating?

By figuring out how to draw in your muscles to remain standing, you're conditioning them, yet additionally working on your command over your body and your perseverance. As per Harvard Clinical School, ice skating will wreck to 200 calories each hour, making it an incredible method for losing or keep up with weight when joined with a solid eating routine.

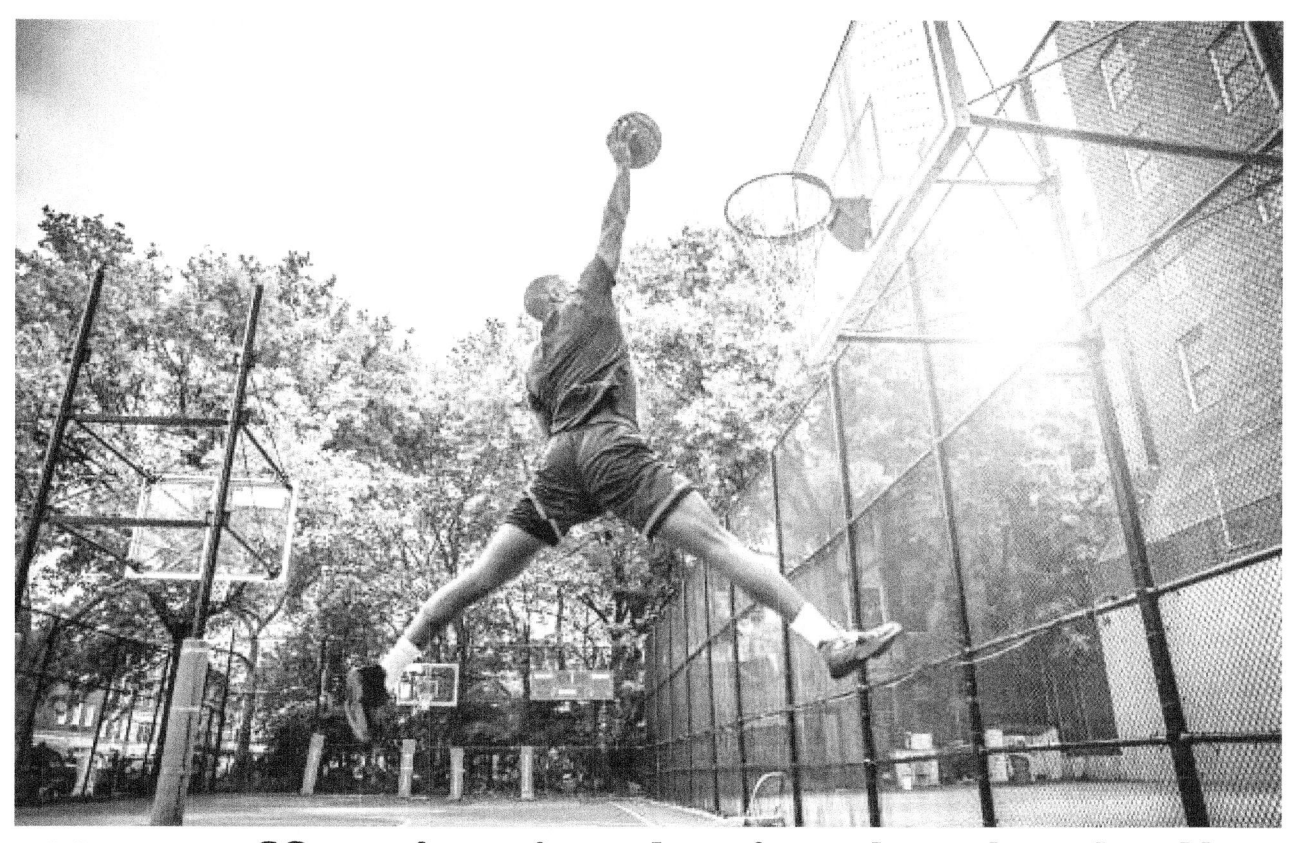

How effective is playing basketball?

Playing b-ball assists with working on engine coordination, adaptability, and perseverance. It additionally empowers speed, readiness, and strength. These abilities are displayed to emphatically affect advancing a sound body weight and empowering more active work, which can upgrade cardiorespiratory wellness and confidence

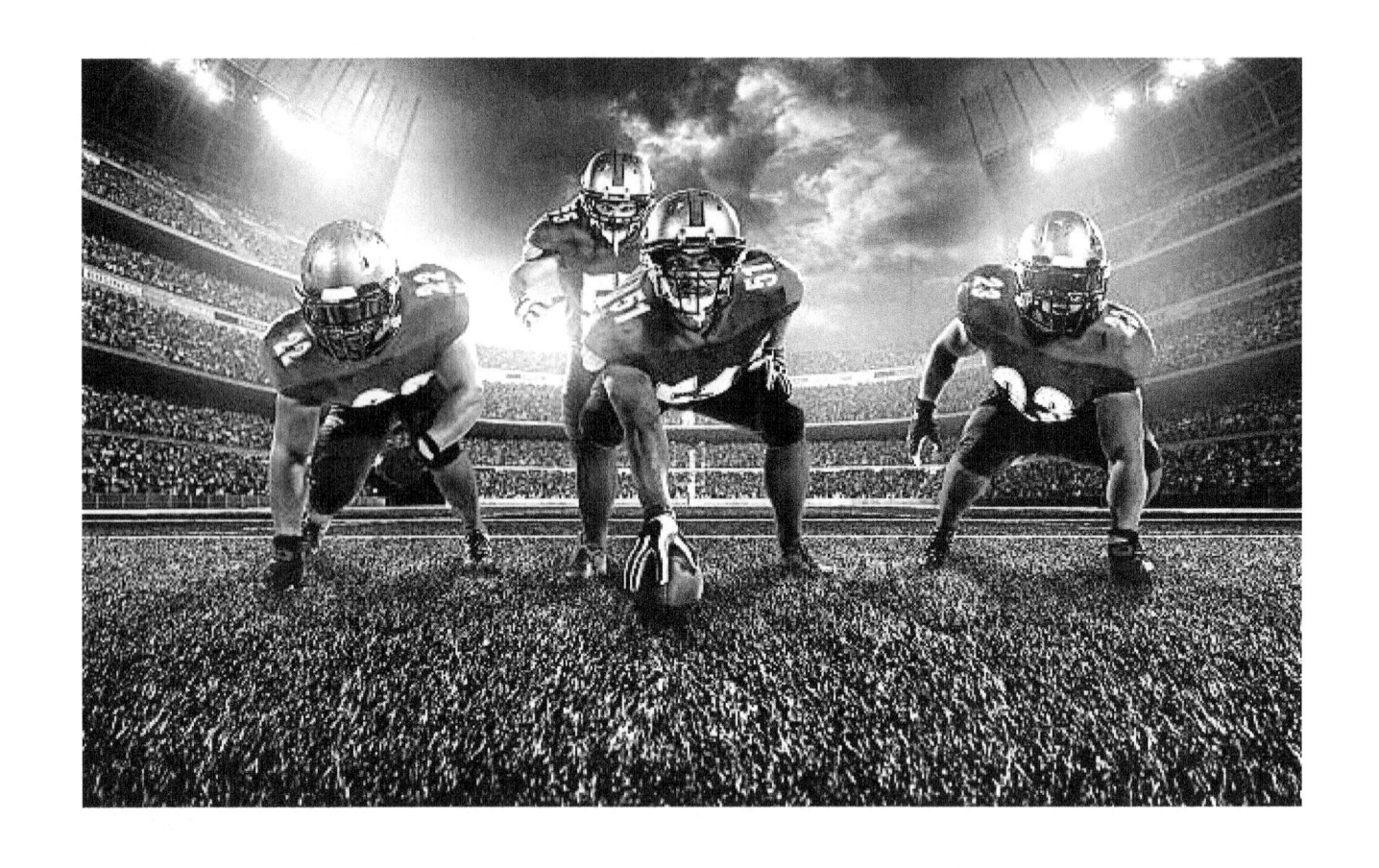

How effective is playing football?

The medical advantages of football include:

Expanding bulk and bone strength in dormant people. Decreasing muscle to fat ratio. Developing fortitude, endurance and speed. Preparing your cerebrum, further developing focus and coordination.

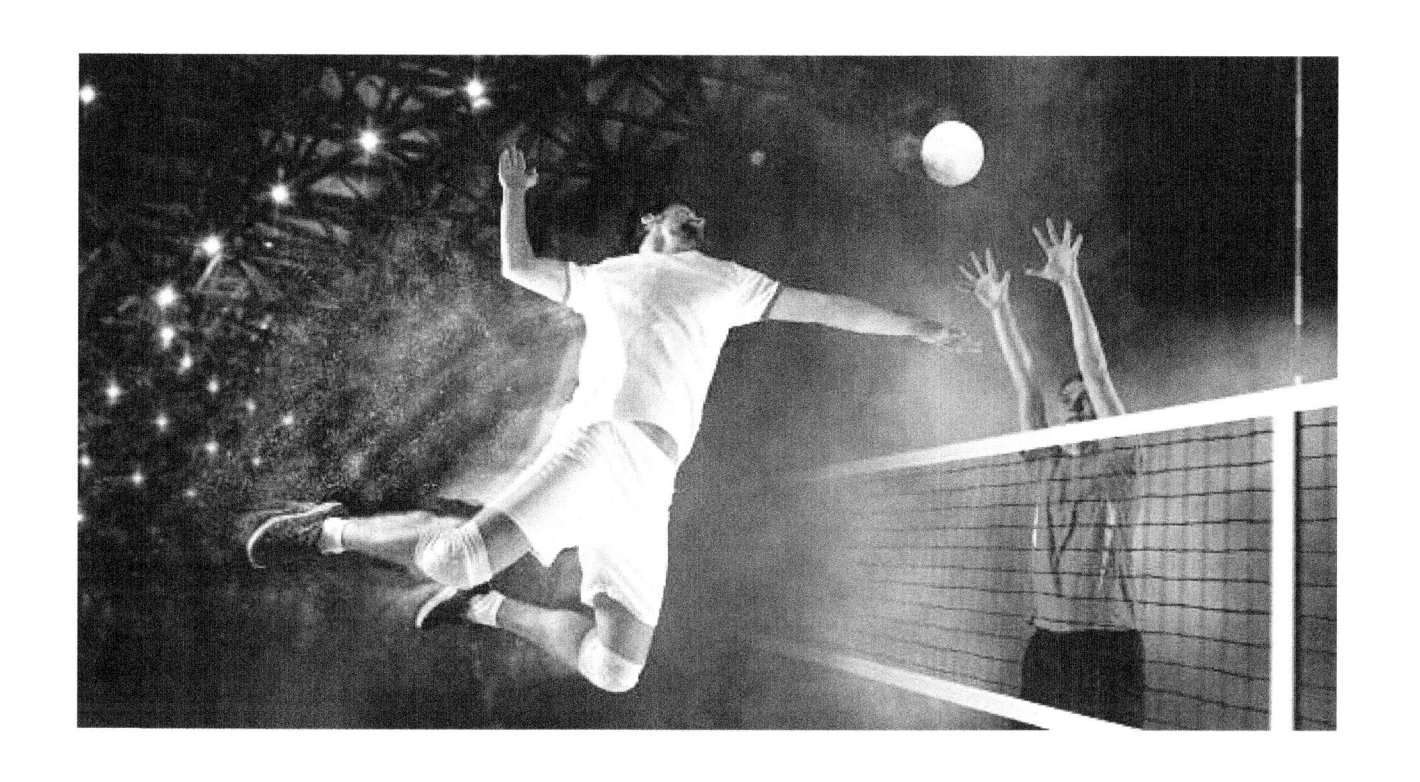

How effective is volleyball?

It can likewise tone and fortify the cardiovascular and respiratory framework. Volleyball can assist with coursing more blood, oxygen, and supplements into the body as well as upgrade your energy levels to further develop your general prosperity. You can likewise foster superior dexterity and quick reflexes.

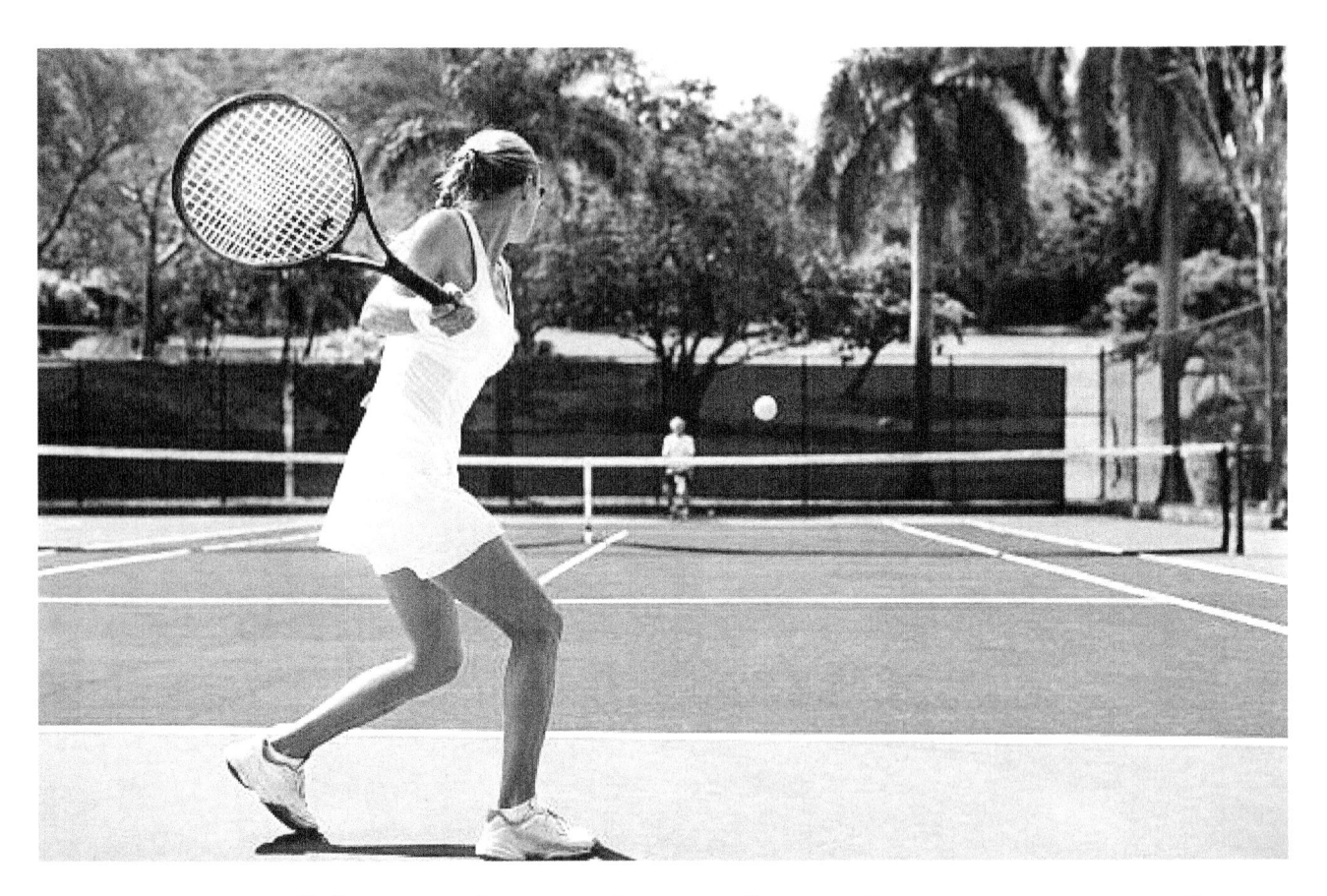

How effective is playing tennis?

Tennis is an incredible cardiovascular activity that works on strong strength, perseverance, equilibrium, coordination, and spryness. Since you really want an accomplice to play a match, it can likewise increment social collaborations. Besides, tennis is a game you can play at whatever stage in life.

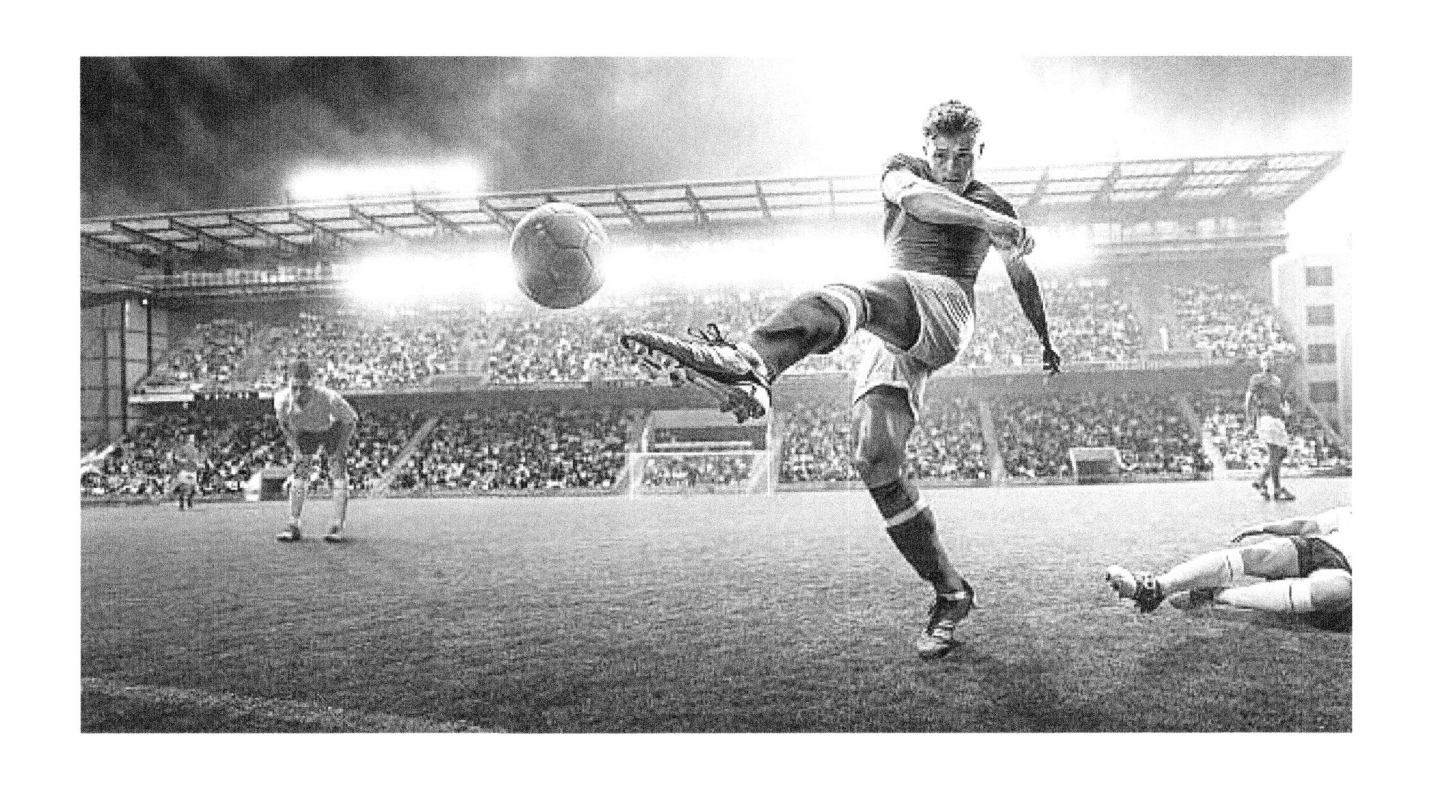

How effective is playing soccer?

Actual Advantages of Playing Soccer. Soccer is perfect for individuals' constitution as it makes you rabbit around a pitch and continually raising your pulse through runs and transport runs. Other than that, it additionally assists you with acquiring muscle, strength, and endurance which assist with injury avoidance and working on your general wellbeing.

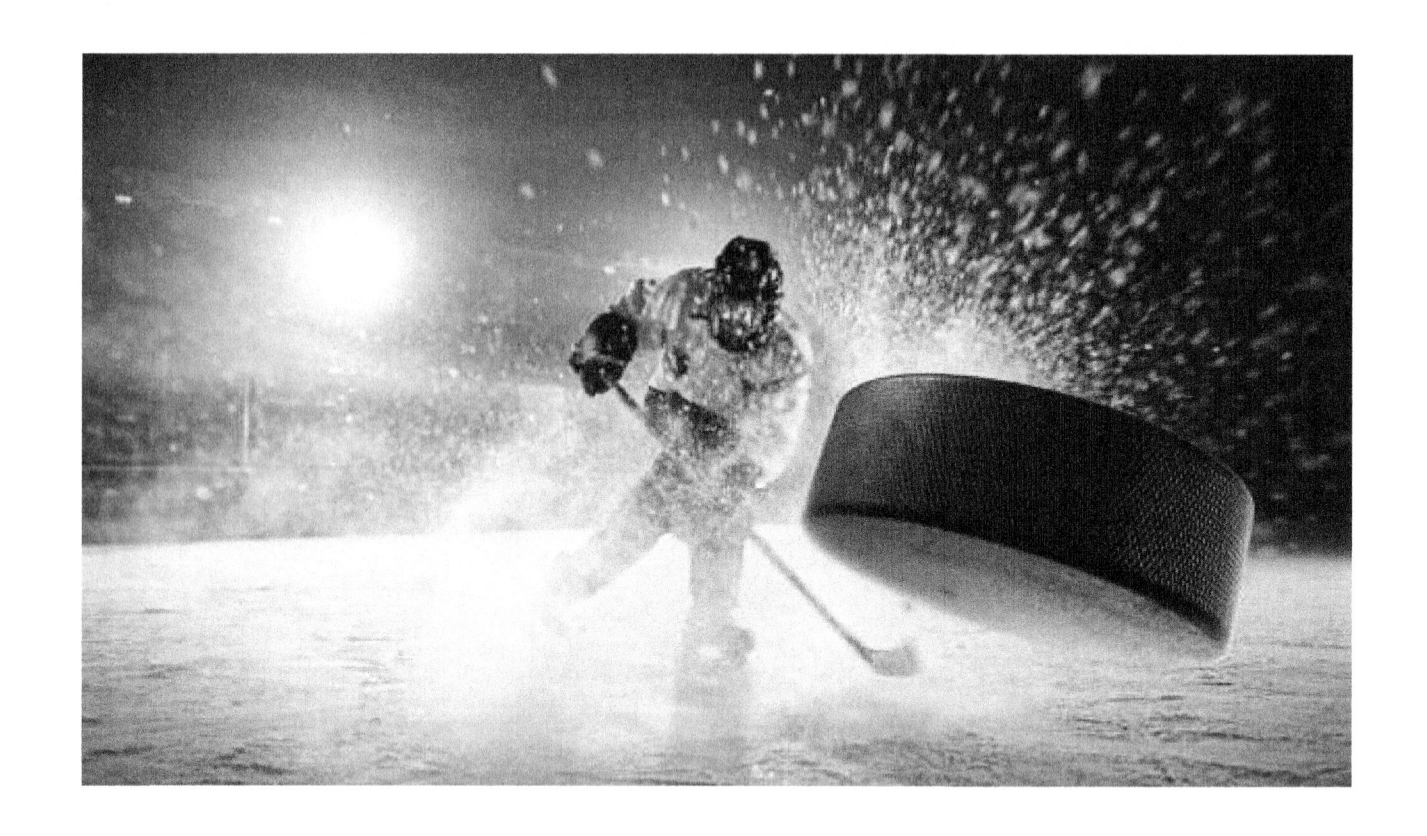

How effective is playing hockey?

What are actual advantages of playing ice hockey?
Hockey is perhaps of all that cardiovascular game you can play. Shifting back and forth among skating and rest (what is known as span preparing in the wellness world) works on the proficiency of the cardiovascular framework, permitting it to rapidly carry oxygen to the muscles more.

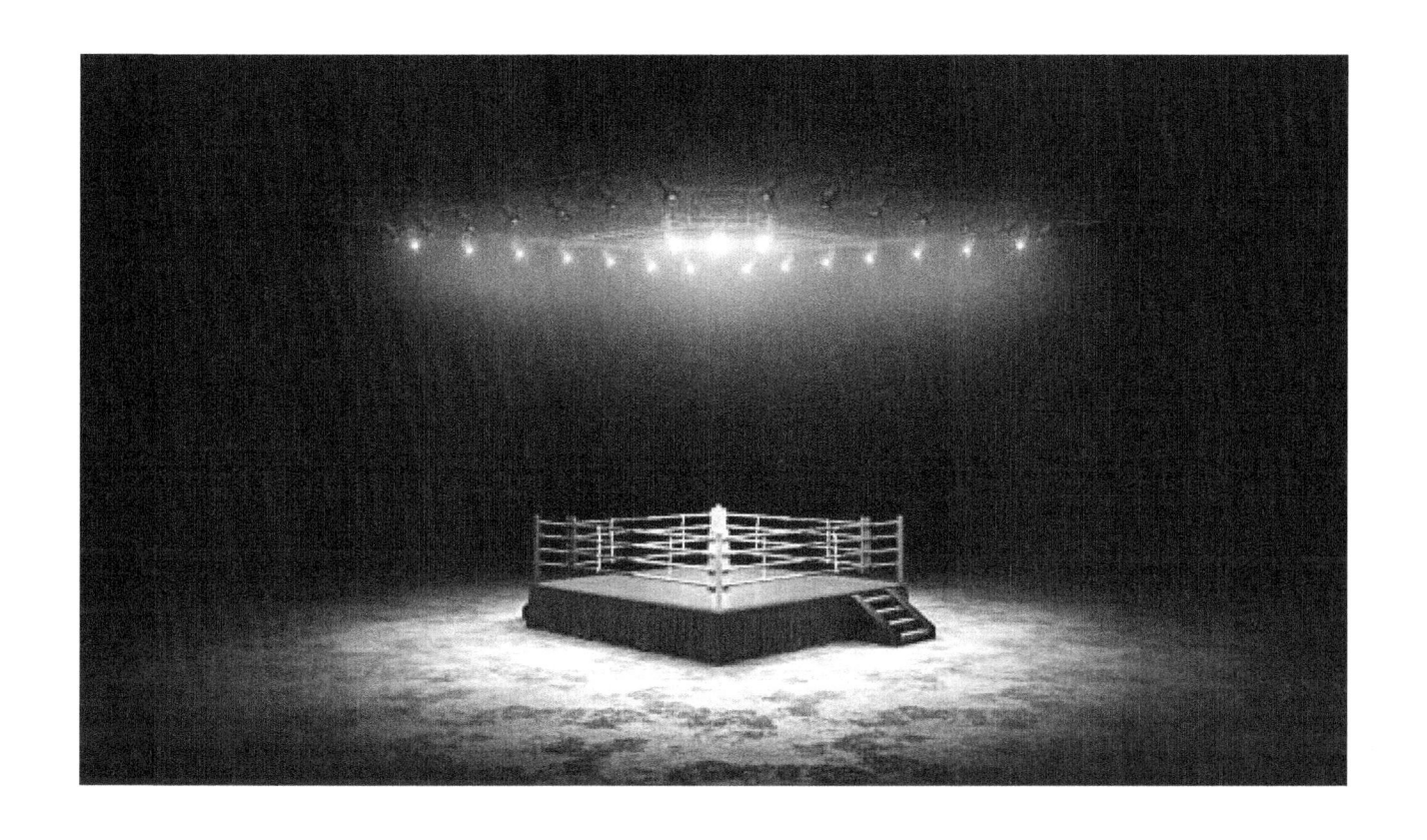

How effective is wrestling?

Wrestling is a profoundly viable type of self-protection. It assists you with associating your striking abilities and your catching skills in a consistent manner. You figure out how to direct whether a battle stays on the feet or on the ground. With Wrestling, you figure out how to utilize strain and control to kill your aggressor.

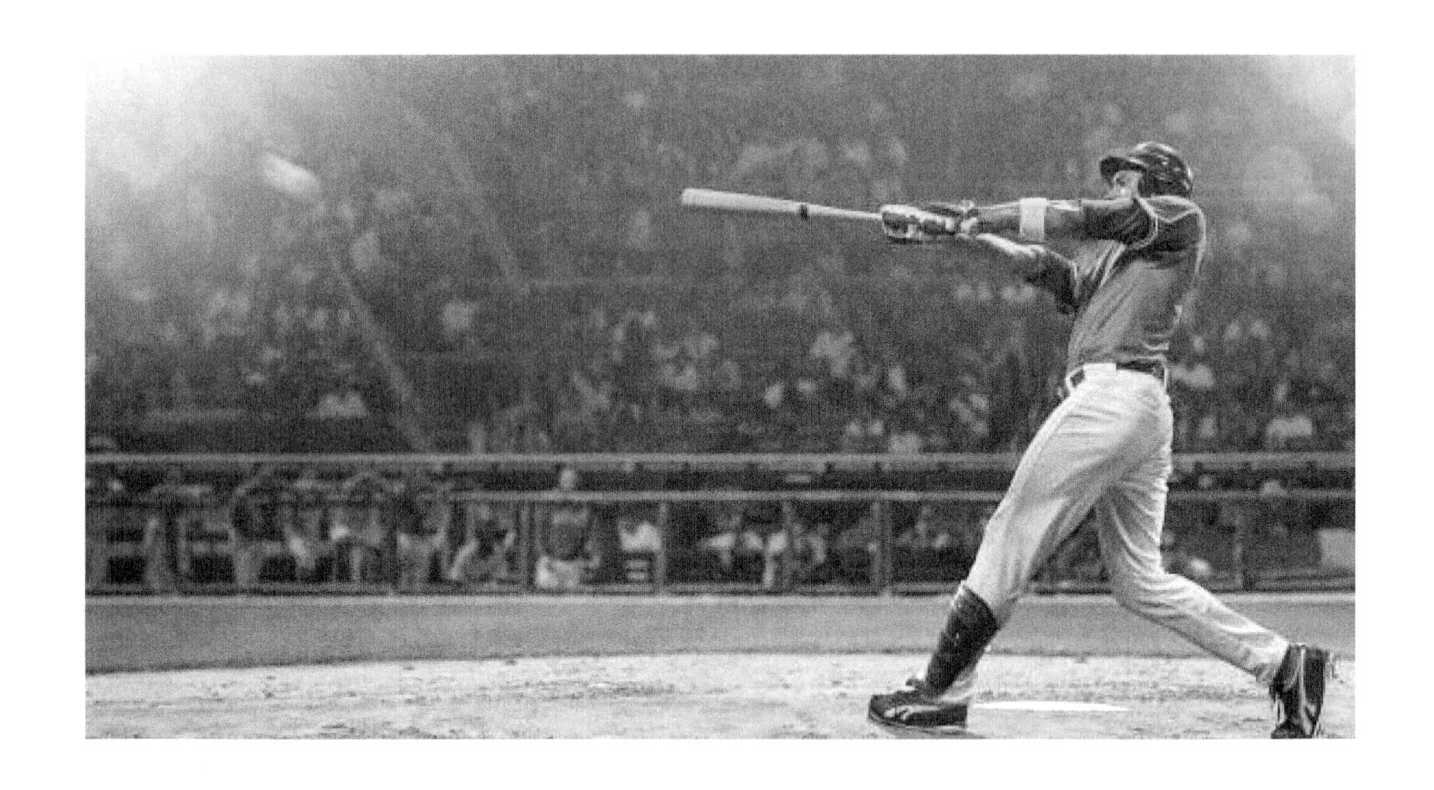

How effective is playing baseball?

Playing baseball develops fortitude in your arms and legs
Holding and swinging a homerun stick and tossing and getting the ball requires utilization of the whole chest area. Certain movements, such as swinging, can likewise construct joint adaptability. Your legs will likewise get an extraordinary exercise.

Printed in Great Britain
by Amazon